Dr.Nowzaradan diet plan book for beginners

Unlock a new You, the effortless route to healthy living and elevated self-esteem easy recipes, the no-fuss diet plan for a complete lifestyle overhaul

Noah Emerson

Table of contents

Chapter 1. Introduction to Dr. Nowzaradan and His Dietary Philosophy

Intro

In the vast world of dieting, where every corner holds a new trend, a superfood, or a miraculous fasting method, it's easy to lose oneself. Everywhere you turn, there's a new promise: a promise of swift weight loss, of chiseled physiques, and of picture-perfect health. However, as the urban population navigating the maze of modern life knows, these fleeting trends often lack a holistic perspective. They focus on the outcome, not the journey. And more often than not, they target the plate, not the person holding it.

This is where our exploration begins, in bustling metropolises, amid the cacophony of clashing ideologies about health, diet, and body image. While diet fads and lifestyle trends come and go, the essence of true health remains consistent: it is a balance of the mind, body, and soul. It is not just about counting calories but understanding their source, their role, and their impact. But where does one start? How does one filter out the noise and grasp the essence of genuine well-being?

Enter Dr. Nowzaradan, a luminary in the domain of weight management and holistic health. But this book, inspired by his philosophies, is not just another addition to the towering stack of recipe books in your kitchen or the countless diet manuals collecting dust on your shelf. Instead, this is an invitation to a journey—a journey that delves deep into the relationship between food, weight, and overall health.

When you look around a modern metropolitan city, you see a reflection of progress, but also of paradoxes. The conveniences of modern urban life, from food delivery apps to escalators, are undeniable. However, these very conveniences have led many astray, distancing them from the roots of a healthy lifestyle. This book seeks to bridge that gap. Rather than offering mere recipes, it aims to impart wisdom—a wisdom that not only educates about the nutritional content of food but its broader implications on our health, well-being, and societal structures.

Just think about it: How often do we eat without thinking? How frequently do we choose a meal based on convenience rather than nutrition? In the rush of city life, amid endless meetings, deadlines, and responsibilities, nutrition often becomes an afterthought, replaced by whatever is quickest or most accessible. But at what cost?

The intention of this book is not to make you renounce your favorite foods or push you into a stringent, joyless eating regime. No. Instead, it endeavors to rekindle a connection—a connection between the food you consume, the body you nourish, and the life you lead. This is not about quick fixes; it's about lasting change. It's about understanding that the kitchen isn't just a place to cook food—it's a sanctuary where health begins.

Origins and Career of Dr. Nowzaradan

In the vast world of health and nutrition, few figures are as instantly recognizable as Dr. Younan Nowzaradan, affectionately known by many as "Dr. Now." Born in Iran in 1944, his early life was filled with both challenges and ambition. With dreams that extended beyond the borders of his birth country, he pursued a path of medicine and quickly became one of the shining stars in the medical community.

His journey to the United States was not just a geographic transition; it was a leap towards global recognition. Completing his medical degree at the University of Tehran in Iran, Dr. Nowzaradan made the courageous decision to move to America, where he completed his surgical internship at St. Johns Hospital in Detroit, Michigan. His subsequent endeavors, especially his residency in cardiovascular surgery at the Texas Heart Institute in Houston, solidified his place as a leading expert in his field.

While many surgeons achieve success by narrowing their focus, Dr. Now's expertise is commendably broad, spanning general and vascular surgery. Yet, what truly distinguishes him is not just the breadth of his knowledge but his specialty in bariatric surgery, which deals with weight loss and its associated conditions. It is a field that's not only technically challenging but deeply intertwined with the psychological and emotional aspects of patient care.

Many might recognize Dr. Nowzaradan from the popular TV series, 'My 600-lb Life,' where he takes on the arduous task of helping morbidly obese individuals reclaim their lives. The show, however, is not just about weight loss surgeries; it's about transforming lives. Dr. Now uses a blend of strict discipline, undeniable expertise, and heartfelt compassion to guide his patients through their weight loss journeys.

Yet, the spotlight of television does not fully capture the essence of Dr. Nowzaradan's career. His medical practice in Houston, Texas, has been a beacon of hope for thousands who have walked through its doors, seeking a better life. His numerous publications and research projects underline the deep commitment he has to his field, always aiming to advance our understanding of obesity and its associated health risks.

An important aspect of Dr. Nowzaradan's approach is his unwavering belief in the interconnection between the mind and body. For him, bariatric surgery isn't a magical solution but a tool – one that must be complemented with mental resolve, dietary discipline, and a supportive environment. He recognizes that each patient is unique, carrying their own stories, struggles, and dreams. And it's in understanding these nuances that Dr. Now crafts his treatment plans, always ensuring they're tailored to individual needs.

Now, one might wonder, what drives a man like Dr. Nowzaradan? Why choose a path that's fraught with such profound emotional and physical challenges? Perhaps it's his innate belief in the human spirit and its capacity to change. Or maybe, it's the countless success stories, the glimmer of happiness in a patient's eyes, or the quiet moments of gratitude that make all the hurdles worthwhile.

Dr. Nowzaradan's journey, from his early days in Iran to the bustling corridors of his clinic in Houston, is not just a testament to his skills as a surgeon but his qualities as a human being. He has become an emblem of hope and transformation in the weight loss community, with a philosophy that's rooted in both scientific rigor and heartfelt compassion.

In the chapters ahead, we will delve deeper into the intricacies of his dietary approach, the pillars of his philosophy, and the actionable steps one can take to embark on a journey toward better health and a more fulfilling life. As we progress, let Dr. Nowzaradan's story be a reminder: change, however challenging, is always within reach.

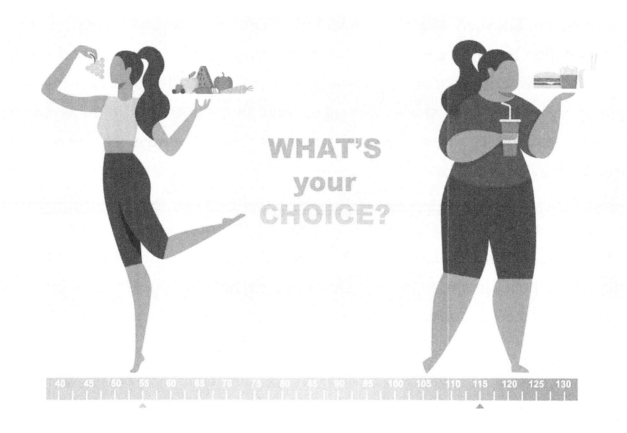

The Importance of Weight and Health

In the tapestry of life, where each thread represents an element of our existence, two strands stand out for their undeniable significance: weight and health. Their intricate dance affects not just the individual, but ripples outward, influencing families, communities, and societies at large. Understanding this interplay, especially in the backdrop of our modern lifestyle, isn't a luxury; it's an imperative.

The bustling streets of metropolitan cities, dotted with skyscrapers and bathed in neon lights, tell a story. It's a narrative of progress, ambition, and ceaseless energy. Yet, beneath this veneer lies another tale, one of long working hours, convenience foods, and reduced physical activity. The urban lifestyle, with all its benefits, has inadvertently set many on a path where weight gain becomes almost an inevitable side effect.

But why does this matter? Isn't weight just a number, a mere reflection of our gravitational interaction with the Earth? At a cursory glance, perhaps. But delve deeper, and it's evident that our weight is a barometer of our overall health.

Our bodies are marvels of engineering, constantly striving to maintain an equilibrium known as homeostasis. Whether it's regulating temperature, pH, or glucose levels, the body's mechanisms work tirelessly. Weight plays into this balance in a myriad of ways.

Firstly, our weight influences our cardiovascular system. Carrying extra pounds means the heart needs to work harder, pumping blood to a larger mass of tissue, potentially leading to elevated blood pressure and increased risks of heart disease.

Musculoskeletal health, too, feels the impact. Our spine, hips, and knees bear the brunt of our daily movements. Add excess weight, and the wear and tear on these joints escalate, often leading to chronic conditions like osteoarthritis.

Yet, the effects aren't just physical. Excess weight has been linked to a plethora of mental health issues. Feelings of inadequacy, societal pressure, and self-esteem challenges can spiral into more severe conditions like depression and anxiety.

However, viewing weight and health solely from an individual lens might be myopic. It's a societal concern. Rising obesity rates strain healthcare systems, with increased hospital admissions and skyrocketing medical costs. Productivity dips as more workers take sick days. Families suffer, watching loved ones grapple with weight-induced health issues.

So, what's the antidote? Surely, in an era marked by technological marvels, there's a solution to the weight conundrum? The reality, as many discover, isn't about finding a magic pill or a revolutionary diet. It's about revisiting the basics, understanding the core principles of nutrition and health, and aligning one's lifestyle accordingly.

Enter figures like Dr. Nowzaradan, who don't just view weight from a surgical or medical perspective but see it as a holistic challenge. For professionals like him, every patient's journey starts with understanding. It's about comprehending that behind every statistic is a real person, with dreams, fears, and aspirations.

For many in metropolitan cities, sandwiched between deadlines and commitments, health often takes a backseat. Fast food replaces wholesome meals, Netflix supersedes gym sessions, and slowly, the pounds creep in. But it's not just about aesthetics or fitting into a particular dress size. It's about life quality, longevity, and the sheer joy of living without the constant shadow of health concerns.

The urban dweller of today needs more than just diet charts or exercise routines. They need a philosophy, an ethos that guides them back to the essentials of health. This isn't about deprivation or stringent rules. It's about understanding, making informed choices, and celebrating the body's potential to heal, rejuvenate, and thrive.

The correlation between weight and health is undeniable. But in this relationship lies hope. Just as weight gain can trigger a cascade of health issues, weight loss, done right, can usher in a renaissance of wellbeing. With guidance, support, and a touch of determination, the journey from weight-ensnared to health-empowered is not just possible; it's waiting.

As we delve deeper into this book, let the principles outlined be more than mere words. Let them be a beacon, illuminating the path to a life marked by vitality, vigor, and the unmatched joy of holistic health.

Conclusion

As we wrap up this introductory chapter, let's step back and reflect. The narrative that unfolds in the subsequent pages is not just about what ingredients to use or how to plate your dish. It is, above all, a guide to understanding. An understanding that health isn't built in a day or with a single meal, but over time, with consistent choices and an awareness of one's body and needs.

Dr. Nowzaradan's philosophy serves as a beacon, shedding light on the often murky waters of diet and health, offering a clearer, more holistic path. A path that respects individuality, cherishes balance, and emphasizes the joy of eating as much as the benefits of nutrition.

This is not just a book; it's a companion for your journey towards a healthier, happier life. As you turn the pages, remember: every chapter, every sentence, every word is a stepping stone towards a lifestyle that celebrates both the pleasure of food and the vitality of good health. Let's embark on this journey together, hand in hand, plate by plate, towards a brighter, healthier future.

Chapter 2. Basics of Dr. Nowzaradan's Diet

Intro

In the vast expanse of dietary information available today, it's easy to be overwhelmed. Every day, a new diet promises miraculous results. Amidst this cacophony, Dr. Nowzaradan's approach emerges as a refreshing voice of reason, grounded not in transient trends but in timeless truths. At the heart of his philosophy lies the understanding of macronutrients and their roles in our diet. As you navigate through this chapter, you'll uncover the essence of these nutrients, with a particular emphasis on the undeniable importance of protein in our daily lives.

Imagine the bustling streets of a metropolitan city – skyscrapers, car horns, coffee shops at every corner, and a relentless pace of life. In such a setting, nourishing our bodies adequately becomes both a challenge and a necessity. Given our urban lifestyle's demands, understanding the basics of nutrition becomes as fundamental as comprehending the rhythms of city life. Much like the foundation of a towering skyscraper, our dietary choices form the bedrock upon which our health is built. And protein, as you'll soon discover, is a central pillar in this foundation.

However, to appreciate protein's role fully, one needs to delve deeper than surface-level knowledge. This chapter aims to be a guiding light, illuminating the multifaceted nature of protein and its impact on our overall well-being. Whether you're someone who's traversed the journey of diets or someone just beginning to understand nutrition's nuances, the insights shared here aim to resonate with your quest for a balanced and fulfilling life.

But why place such emphasis on protein? Is it merely a dietary component, or does it play a larger role in the grand tapestry of our well-being? The subsequent sections will answer these questions, marrying science with everyday experiences, making the subject matter both relatable and rooted in evidence.

Moreover, in the urban sprawl, where convenience often trumps nutrition, understanding protein's importance can be a transformative experience. It can empower you to make conscious choices, to sift through the myriad options available, and to embrace a diet that harmoniously complements your lifestyle.

The journey with Dr. Nowzaradan's philosophy is not about drastic changes or unrealistic expectations. It's about equipping oneself with knowledge, understanding one's body, and recognizing the silent, profound ways in which nutrients like protein impact our daily lives. As we delve into this chapter, let us embark on this enlightening journey together, guided by science, inspired by real-life experiences, and anchored by Dr. Nowzaradan's wisdom.

Calories and Nutritional Balance: The Foundation of Holistic Health

In a bustling urban world, filled with fast-food joints at every corner and convenience foods lining supermarket shelves, understanding the genuine meaning behind the terms 'calories' and 'nutrition' can feel like deciphering a foreign language. We've all been there—picking up a pack of cookies that boasts "Only 100 calories!" or a bottle of soda that proudly declares "Zero calories!" But do these calorie counts genuinely serve our health? Do they paint the full picture of our nutritional needs?

Before diving into Dr. Nowzaradan's philosophy, let's embark on a short journey to understand what calories truly are. Contrary to popular belief, calories aren't malevolent entities lurking in your food, ready to add inches to your waistline. Instead, they're units of energy. Each calorie represents the energy required to raise the temperature of one gram of water by one degree Celsius. Simply put, calories are the fuel that keeps the magnificent machine called the human body running.

But here's the catch: not all calories are created equal. Think of your body as a high-end vehicle. Just as you wouldn't pour low-grade gasoline into a luxury car, you shouldn't fuel your body with empty-calorie foods. A candy bar and an avocado might have the same number of calories, but their nutritional profiles are worlds apart.

To appreciate the depth of Dr. Nowzaradan's philosophy, we must first acknowledge that eating is not merely an act of ingesting calories. It's about nourishing our bodies. Every bite we take can either contribute to our health or detract from it. Imagine for a moment two plates. On one plate, you have a sugary donut, and on the other, a medley of fresh fruits. Both plates may offer a similar caloric value, but their impacts on our health are diametrically opposed.

The donut, brimming with sugars and unhealthy fats, offers instant energy— a short-lived spike in blood sugar, followed by an inevitable crash. On the other hand, the fruits provide not only energy in the form of natural sugars but also vital vitamins, minerals, and fibers. While the donut might appeal to your taste buds momentarily, the fruits cater to your body's long-term health and well-being.

Nutritional balance is a phrase that's often thrown around but rarely understood in its entirety. It's not about meeting a specific caloric goal or adhering strictly to the ratios on a nutrition label. Instead, it's about understanding our body's needs and answering its call for nourishment.

Every individual's nutritional needs differ based on their age, gender, activity level, and overall health. For instance, a professional athlete's dietary requirements would differ vastly from those of an office worker. Hence, there's no "one-size-fits-all" diet.

Dr. Nowzaradan's approach isn't about strict calorie counting or depriving oneself. It's about achieving a balance—knowing when to indulge, when to hold back, and understanding the ripple effects of our dietary choices. It's about recognizing that a calorie isn't just a calorie; it's a potential powerhouse of nutrition.

City life, with its endless array of dining options, can be both a boon and a bane. The key lies in making informed choices. Let's say you're at a metropolitan café, facing a menu. The grilled chicken salad and the creamy pasta have a similar calorie count. Yet, one offers lean protein and an array of veggies, while the other is dense with saturated fats.

Such scenarios underscore the importance of discerning not just how many calories a dish offers, but where those calories come from. Dr. Nowzaradan's philosophy emphasizes this discernment, urging us to view food not just as sustenance but as a symphony of nutrients, working in harmony to sustain, heal, and energize our bodies.

As we venture further into the nuances of Dr. Nowzaradan's diet, remember this foundational principle: calories and nutrition are intertwined, but they're not synonymous. In the grand tapestry of health, calories form the threads, while nutrition determines the pattern. In the upcoming chapters, we'll delve deeper into making sense of these threads, guiding you to weave a life filled with vitality, balance, and joy.

The Importance of Protein in the Diet

When most of us think of protein, visions of muscle-bound gym-goers consuming protein shakes come to mind. But the significance of protein transcends the walls of any gym. For the everyday individual navigating the hustle and bustle of city life, understanding protein is pivotal for more reasons than we might initially reckon.

At its core, protein is a macronutrient, a fundamental pillar of our diet. Comprised of amino acids, often dubbed as the body's building blocks, proteins play a quintessential role in repairing tissues, making enzymes, and synthesizing hormones. Whether you're a stay-at-home parent chasing after kids or an executive managing a bustling metropolitan office, your body requires protein not just for strength, but for overall functionality.

City life, especially in a metropolitan setting, is often paradoxical. With the comforts of modern living come the challenges of sedentary lifestyles. Amid this backdrop, managing one's weight becomes not just about vanity, but a quest for holistic well-being.

Here's where protein packs a punch. Consuming protein-rich foods can induce a sensation of fullness, curbing those sudden hunger pangs and reducing overall calorie intake. When you're satiated, you're less likely to reach for that conveniently placed sugary snack. Moreover, the body expends more energy to process proteins compared to fats or carbs, giving a subtle boost to your metabolism.

Life in the urban jungle can be relentless. The demands of work, the challenges of navigating traffic, the social pressures of maintaining an 'image' all of it requires stamina, resilience, and mental agility. Proteins play a silent yet formidable role in aiding these endeavors.

For instance, certain amino acids derived from protein-rich foods are precursors to neurotransmitters responsible for mood regulation. The hustle and drive of city life, while exhilarating, can also be mentally draining. Ensuring adequate protein intake can be a game-changer in managing stress and emotional well-being.

The beauty of protein is its versatility. From a juicy steak to a hearty lentil soup, from a piece of grilled fish to a soy stir-fry, the sources of protein are vast and varied. This diversity ensures that irrespective of one's dietary choices—be it meat-lover, vegetarian, or vegan there's no dearth of options to meet protein needs.

Moreover, with the increasing culinary innovations in metropolitan cities, there's a delightful fusion of taste and nutrition. It's entirely feasible to enjoy a protein-rich meal that's not just nutritionally robust but also a treat to the taste buds. In the heart of the city, one can find both traditional protein-rich dishes and modern interpretations that align with Dr. Nowzaradan's philosophy.

One of the most pervasive myths is that only those who engage in intense physical activity need substantial protein. Nothing could be further from the truth. While athletes might have heightened protein needs, every individual regardless of their level of physical activity requires protein for basic bodily functions.

Think about it. The very act of living, of breathing, of thinking, requires cellular activities that are underpinned by proteins. The wear and tear our bodies undergo, even without strenuous activity, necessitates repair and regeneration, roles in which protein is indispensable.

Embracing the importance of protein isn't about jumping on a new diet trend. It's about recognizing and respecting our body's innate needs. In the grand tapestry of life, especially in the vibrant yet challenging milieu of city living, protein emerges not just as a nutrient, but as a steadfast ally.

Dr. Nowzaradan's emphasis on protein isn't a mere dietary whim. It's rooted in science, in understanding the human body, and in acknowledging the myriad roles protein plays in our daily lives.

As we meander through the maze of modern living, armed with the wisdom of dietary choices, may we always remember the profound simplicity of protein's power. Not just as a macronutrient, but as a companion in our journey toward well-being, vitality, and a life fully lived.

Conclusion

As we draw this chapter to a close, let's take a moment to reflect on the journey we've traversed together. The intricate world of protein, often relegated to the confines of gym conversations, has been unveiled in its entirety, revealing its multifaceted role in our well-being. In the hustle and bustle of city life, amidst the challenges of urban living, protein emerges not just as a dietary component, but as a trusted ally in our quest for health and vitality.

The importance of protein in Dr. Nowzaradan's diet is no accident. It's a testament to the nutrient's undeniable significance, echoing centuries of nutritional wisdom. Armed with this knowledge, you are now poised to make informed dietary choices, ones that resonate with your unique lifestyle and health aspirations.

Yet, the journey doesn't end here. As with any profound understanding, the insights gleaned from this chapter beckon to be integrated into our daily lives. They urge us to be conscious consumers, to view our plates not just as a medley of foods, but as a mosaic of nutrients, each with its unique story and significance.

In the grand narrative of health and well-being, protein plays a starring role. But its true magic lies not just in understanding its importance but in weaving it seamlessly into our daily lives. As we move forward, may we do so with a renewed appreciation for this remarkable nutrient, guided by Dr. Nowzaradan's wisdom, and inspired by the promise of a healthier, more vibrant life.

Chapter 3. The Right Mindset for Success

Intro

In the grand theatre of life, our aspirations play the lead roles. They dictate our actions, shape our paths, and become the narratives we share with the world. In a metropolitan city, amidst the blaring horns, the towering skyscrapers, and the never-ending hustle, everyone is on a journey, chasing a dream. While the goals might vary – a promotion, a house, or in the context of this chapter, a healthier self – the underlying essence remains constant: the desire for success. But what determines this success? Is it merely hard work, luck, or resources? While these elements play their parts, at the heart of every triumph lies a crucial ingredient: the right mindset.

The urban jungle teaches us many lessons. It mirrors life's ups and downs, its unpredictability, and its endless potential. Yet, one lesson stands out – the importance of perspective. In the realm of personal health and fitness, this perspective translates to our mindset. Two individuals might have the same goal, access to identical resources, and even similar backgrounds. Yet, one succeeds while the other falters. The differentiator? Their mindset. This chapter dives deep into the labyrinth of our psyche, exploring the mental and behavioral challenges one faces when embarking on a journey towards better health and how to set realistic and measurable goals that pave the way for lasting success.

Addressing Mental and Behavioral Challenges

Navigating the winding road of dietary transformation is often less about the food we consume and more about the mindset that fuels our journey. While understanding the fundamentals of nutrition and following a structured plan are crucial, tackling the intricate web of our mental and behavioral challenges can be the real game-changer. For in these challenges lie deeply rooted habits, beliefs, and perceptions that, more often than not, steer our decisions, actions, and outcomes.

For many, the urban milieu of metropolitan life comes with its unique set of mental pressures. The relentless hustle, constant comparisons, and the incessant chase for perfection can cultivate a mental environment rife with self-doubt, anxiety, and unrealistic expectations. While these pressures can sometimes act as motivators, pushing us to strive for better, they can also become burdens, weighing down our aspirations with the chains of negative self-perception.

Imagine being in a room filled with mirrors. Every reflection shows a different version of you. Some reflections might magnify your perceived flaws, while others might diminish your strengths. Such is the nature of our thoughts. They can distort reality, leading us to see ourselves not as we truly are, but as fragmented reflections shaped by external judgments and internal fears.

So, how does one break free from this maze of distorted reflections? The first step is recognizing the existence of unhealthy behaviors. These behaviors might manifest as binge eating after a stressful day, skipping meals to "compensate" for perceived overindulgence, or constantly seeking validation from scales and measuring tapes.

For the 45-year-old executive, it might be the habitual consumption of fast food because he equates long hours at work with deserving unhealthy rewards. For the 32-year-old artist, it might be the irregular eating patterns, stemming from erratic work schedules and a belief that creativity thrives on chaos. For the 55-year-old mother, it might be the sacrifice of her dietary needs, placing her family's preferences above her own health.

Dr. Nowzaradan emphasizes the intricate link between our mental well-being and physical health. One cannot thrive without the other. This understanding is pivotal. When we begin to see our dietary choices not as isolated actions but as reflections of our mental state, we gain a clearer perspective on the root causes of our challenges.

A deep dive into our behavioral patterns might reveal that the late-night snacking is less about hunger and more about loneliness. The skipped breakfast might not be due to a lack of time but a manifestation of self-neglect. And the overindulgence during social events might be less about the food and more about seeking comfort in familiarity amidst the chaos of social anxiety.

To navigate this journey of self-discovery and transformation, two tools are indispensable: awareness and compassion. Awareness requires us to be present, to observe our actions and emotions without judgment, and to understand the triggers that lead to specific behaviors. It's about catching yourself in the act, understanding the 'why' behind the action, and gently guiding yourself towards healthier choices.

Compassion, on the other hand, is about extending kindness to oneself. In a world where we're often our harshest critics, showing ourselves the same empathy we offer to others can be revolutionary. It means acknowledging that slip-ups are part of the journey, that every day won't be perfect, and that's okay. It's about viewing every challenge not as a setback but as an opportunity for growth.

Embarking on a journey of dietary transformation is as much an inward journey as it is outward. While the foods we consume play a pivotal role, the thoughts we nurture, the beliefs we hold, and the behaviors we exhibit shape the trajectory of our journey. By addressing our mental and behavioral challenges, by understanding their origins and their impacts, we empower ourselves to make lasting changes. Changes that are not just about the reflection in the mirror but about the essence of who we are and who we aspire to be.

Setting Realistic and Measurable Goals

In the heart of any metropolitan city, the hum of ambition is as ubiquitous as the skyline that stretches towards the horizon. Everywhere you turn, someone's setting a goal, be it in their career, personal life, or health journey. Yet, amidst these sprawling aspirations, one aspect often eludes us – the art of setting realistic and measurable goals.

In an era of instant gratification and highlight reels, it's easy to get lost in the labyrinth of colossal expectations. The stories of overnight successes, drastic transformations, and fairy-tale outcomes fill our screens. But the truth, as many discover often too late, is that sustainable change requires time, patience, and an adherence to reality.

Imagine standing at the base of a skyscraper. Your aim is to reach the top. Would you attempt to leap to the pinnacle in one bound? Certainly not. Instead, you'd find the elevator or the stairs and ascend one floor at a time. Such should be the approach to our goals.

Metropolitan cities, with their pace and persona, inadvertently cultivate myths. "Sarah lost 20 pounds in a month!" or "Mike transformed his life in a week!" These stories, though occasionally true, are exceptions, not norms. When setting goals, it's paramount to sift the facts from fiction.

Every individual's journey is unique. The metabolic rate, genetic makeup, daily routines, and even stress levels play intricate roles in our health endeavors. While Sarah's story is commendable, it might not be applicable to everyone. It's essential to recognize and respect one's own pace and path.

Once we anchor our aspirations in reality, the next step is to ensure they're measurable. It's one thing to say, "I want to feel better," and another to state, "I aim to walk 10,000 steps every day." The latter offers clarity, direction, and an end point to assess progress.

In the vibrant avenues of city life, where every second count, having quantifiable goals can be the beacon that guides through the fog of distractions. It provides a tangible metric, a touchpoint to return to when the journey becomes overwhelming or confusing.

Setting a measurable goal doesn't necessarily mean it has to be vast or intimidating. In fact, the most effective goals often are the ones broken down into smaller, achievable tasks. If the ultimate aim is to lose 50 pounds, start with aiming for 5. Celebrate that victory, then move to the next.

The bustling streets of urban environments often echo with the adage, "Slow and steady wins the race." This principle, age-old yet timeless, holds profound wisdom. Every significant achievement is but a summation of numerous minor victories.

Setting goals that are both realistic and measurable has profound psychological benefits. Every time you achieve a mini-goal, the brain releases dopamine, a neurotransmitter associated with pleasure, learning, and motivation. This not only makes you feel good but also propels you to persevere.

For instance, John, a 40-year-old urban professional, aimed to run a marathon. Instead of focusing on the 26.2 miles from the get-go, he set monthly targets. First, it was running a mile without stopping, then 5k, 10k, and so forth. Each accomplishment fortified his belief and fueled his journey forward.

However, a word of caution. While ambition is admirable, overambition can be treacherous. It's the overzealous leap for the stars without preparing for the journey that often leads to injuries, burnouts, and disillusionment.

In the context of health and fitness, overambition might manifest as extreme diets, over-exercising, or setting unattainable standards. While the initial results might seem promising, the long-term repercussions can be detrimental.

In the vibrant tapestry of urban life, amidst aspirations and ambitions, carving out a space for one's own unique journey is both an art and a science. It requires introspection, a touch of realism, and a dash of ambition.

Setting realistic and measurable goals is not about curbing one's dreams. It's about paving a sustainable path towards them. It's about recognizing that in the marathon of life, it's the steady steps, taken with awareness and consistency, that lead to the most gratifying destinations. Remember, every skyscraper, no matter how tall, is built one brick at a time.

Conclusion

In our pursuit of better health, we often look outside – the latest diet trend, the most advanced gym, or the newest health gadget. Yet, the most potent tool lies within us – our mindset. The cityscape, with its undying spirit and relentless pace, serves as a constant reminder of human potential. But it also subtly underscores the significance of the journey over the destination. The roads we traverse, the choices we make, and the challenges we overcome define our story more than the eventual outcome.

As we conclude this chapter, remember that your health journey, much like life in a metropolitan setting, will be filled with unexpected turns, roadblocks, and sometimes, detours. But with the right mindset – one that's rooted in reality yet optimistic, one that sets measurable milestones yet celebrates every small victory – you'll not only navigate these challenges but also thrive amidst them.

Chapter 4.Meal Planning: What to Eat and What to Avoid

Intro

In the busy metropolis that is modern life, every street corner offers a tantalizing choice, every alley a culinary adventure waiting to be explored. This bustling cityscape, much like our daily lives, presents a myriad of options. However, just as in a sprawling urban setting, not every turn we take aligns with the destination we have in mind.

Have you ever found yourself lost in a city, despite having a map in hand? That's because cities, much like our dietary paths, are complicated. The flashing neon lights of fast-food chains can momentarily overshadow the soft glow of a health-conscious bistro just around the corner. The alluring scent of a bakery might divert us from the fresh aroma of a salad bar a few steps ahead. And much like the city's pulse, our dietary choices are influenced by external factors: the rush of a deadline, the comfort of old habits, the tug of cravings, or even the persuasion of peers.

Imagine for a moment that this chapter is your GPS, and your goal is to navigate the city without getting lost, ensuring that each stop adds value to your journey. The city's streets and avenues are the countless food choices you encounter each day, and the GPS voice guiding you is Dr. Nowzaradan's wisdom. He's here to help you understand which turns to take and which to bypass for a healthier, more nourishing life.

To traverse any city effectively, you must first know its layout, its landmarks, and its less desirable districts. The foods we choose to ingest and those we decide to limit or avoid entirely are much like these urban elements. Some choices set the foundation for a thriving, vibrant life, just as iconic structures and parks do for a city. On the other hand, some foods, while initially tempting, may hinder our journey toward our desired destination, mirroring the city's dead-ends and risky areas.

But fear not. With the right guidance, anyone can become a seasoned traveler, effortlessly navigating the city's streets, making choices that enhance the journey rather than detract from it. As we delve deeper into this chapter, we'll uncover the secrets of the metropolis of meal planning, ensuring that every choice, every turn, takes us closer to our desired destination.

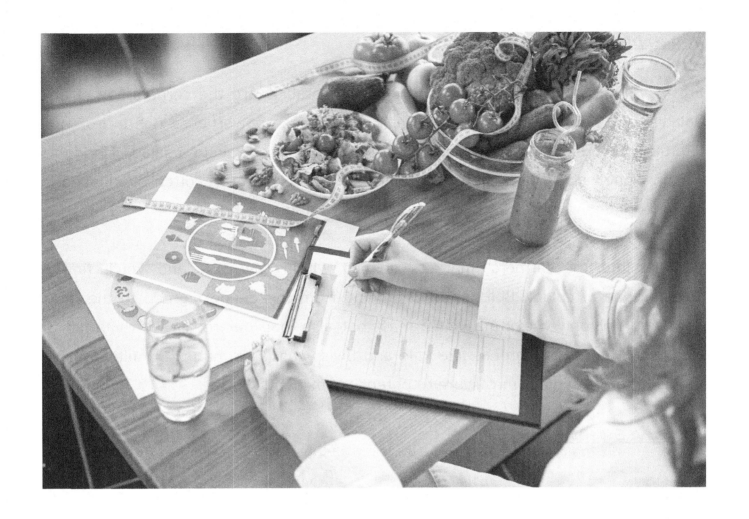

List of allowed foods

Within the sprawling city, in every nook and cranny of its ever-expanding expanse, there exists a fascinating juxtaposition. Just as architectural masterpieces stand alongside ancient structures, embodying the city's history and future, our dietary choices can also reflect the old and the new. For those on a journey towards a healthier self, it's essential to discern which foods represent the building blocks of our desired future and which ones echo past habits best left behind.

Vegetables: Nature's Bounty

Fresh, vibrant, and teeming with nutrients, vegetables are the cornerstone of any balanced diet. Consider the versatile spinach, a green powerhouse rich in iron and vitamins. Whether sautéed in a dash of olive oil or tossed raw in a salad, it brings a wealth of nutrients to our plates. Similarly, the humble carrot, often overlooked in gourmet kitchens, offers a boost of vitamin A, vital for eye health.

Venture into the farmers' markets nestled within the city, and you'll find a kaleidoscope of colors. Bell peppers, ranging from the deepest green to the most fiery red, not only provide a visual feast but also load our meals with vitamin C. Meanwhile, dark leafy greens like kale and Swiss chard are nature's multivitamins, providing everything from calcium to potent antioxidants.

Fruits: A Sweet Affair

While it's easy to reach out for that candy bar during a mid-afternoon slump, imagine replacing it with nature's candy instead. Fruits, in all their natural sweetness, are not just treats for our taste buds but also for our health. Take the blueberry, for example. This tiny, almost unassuming fruit, is a powerhouse of antioxidants. It fights off free radicals and protects our heart.

Then there's the apple, sometimes dubbed the 'miracle food'. Available in various shades and flavors, from the tart Granny Smith to the sweet Honeycrisp, apples are dietary staples that keep the doctor at bay, quite literally!

Proteins: Building Strength from Within

In a city that thrives on energy and momentum, protein is the dietary equivalent of that dynamism. It builds and repairs our muscles, ensuring we're always ready for the next challenge. Legumes like lentils, chickpeas, and beans are not only protein-rich but also packed with fiber, aiding digestion.

Fish, especially fatty varieties like salmon, mackerel, and sardines, are not only delicious but are also teeming with omega-3 fatty acids. These essential fats protect our heart, boost brain health, and even impart a radiant glow to our skin.

Whole Grains: The Unsung Heroes

In a world of dietary fads, whole grains stand tall and unyielding. They have graced our plates for centuries, and with good reason. Quinoa, for instance, once considered the 'gold of the Incas', is a complete protein, boasting all nine essential amino acids. Brown rice, while a staple in many households, offers more than just satiety. It's a source of several vital minerals, including manganese, selenium, and phosphorus.

Dairy and Alternatives: Balancing Tradition and Innovation

Whether you're a purist, reaching out for a glass of milk, or a culinary explorer, sipping on almond or soy milk, this category offers both comfort and novelty. Yogurts, especially the Greek variety, are protein-rich and can be a canvas for flavors, from the sweetness of honey to the tang of fresh berries.

Every meal, much like the city's skyline, is a symphony of choices. The buildings, old and new, tell stories of time, while our plates, filled with a mix of traditional and modern foods, narrate tales of our health journey. As we navigate the myriad of options, remember that every bite counts. It's not just about satiating hunger; it's about nourishing the soul. As you stand at the crossroads of dietary choices, let this list guide you. Here's to making choices that resonate with our health goals, echoing through the vibrant alleyways of our magnificent city, and our equally magnificent bodies.

Foods to avoid or limit

Navigating through the metropolitan culinary scene is much like traversing through the city itself. The wide boulevards brimming with cafes, bars, and restaurants are a testament to the city's ever-evolving palate. But as all city-dwellers know, not every alleyway is safe, and not every dish on the menu is beneficial for our health goals. With the modern rush and our ever-busy lives, it's easy to be swayed by the glitz and glamor of fast food neon signs or the intoxicating aroma of freshly baked sugary treats. But it's crucial to discern which choices pave the way for our goals and which ones lead to detours.

Processed Foods: The Mirages of the Culinary World

There's a reason why window displays at fast-food joints are tantalizingly designed. Much like the flashy billboards in Times Square, they're meant to draw you in. However, beneath the facade often lies a plethora of additives, preservatives, and unhealthy fats. Processed foods, with their high salt and sugar content, may satisfy our immediate cravings but have long-term health implications. Think of it as the city's traffic – momentarily thrilling, but often leading to delays and detours in our health journey.

Sugary Beverages: A Sweet Trap

Walking down a city street on a sweltering summer day, an icy cold soda might seem like the perfect escape. But these beverages, with their high fructose corn syrup and empty calories, are akin to the city's potholes – often unseen but causing significant disruptions. Over time, these drinks can lead to weight gain, tooth decay, and spikes in blood sugar levels. A life lived large needs water, herbal teas, and natural juices to stay genuinely refreshed.

Trans Fats: Hidden Dangers

Much like the alleyways that are best avoided after dark, trans fats in our food can pose dangers that aren't immediately apparent. Found in many fried foods, baked goods, and snacks, these artificial fats can raise bad cholesterol and lower the good kind, increasing the risk of heart diseases. It's the culinary equivalent of the city's smog – not immediately visible but affecting our health with prolonged exposure.

Red and Processed Meats: A Delicate Balance

The aroma of a barbecue on a summer evening can evoke memories and tantalize our senses. And while meats can be a source of essential proteins and nutrients, it's crucial to tread cautiously, especially with red and processed varieties. Excessive consumption can be associated with health risks. So, savor them occasionally, like the city's rare but cherished sunsets, rather than making them a daily spectacle.

Refined Grains: Stripping Away Goodness

Modern processing often strips grains of their natural goodness. Refined grains, like white bread and pasta, have lost much of their fiber, vitamins, and minerals. They're the city's overcrowded tourist spots – initially appealing, but lacking the genuine essence. Instead, whole grains offer a more authentic, nourishing experience.

Alcohol: Moderation is Key

The city's nightlife, with its glitzy bars and clubs, is a significant draw for many. Likewise, a glass of wine or a pint of beer can be a delightful way to unwind. However, just as one wouldn't spend every night partying till dawn, it's essential to limit alcohol intake. Excessive consumption can lead to a range of health issues, from liver problems to an increased risk of certain cancers.

Every city, with its blend of historic landmarks and modern skyscrapers, has areas best explored and others best avoided. Similarly, our dietary choices have their landmarks – foods that nourish, energize, and heal. But they also have pitfalls, foods that might seem appealing in the moment but can steer us away from our health goals.

As we journey towards a healthier self, let's navigate our meals with the same caution and discernment we'd use while exploring a new city. Let's cherish the landmarks, tread cautiously around the pitfalls, and remember: every choice, every bite, every sip shapes the landscape of our health. In this bustling city of life, let's choose pathways that lead us to vibrant health, radiant energy, and a zest for life.

Conclusions

As we wrap up this exploration into the heart of dietary choices, it's essential to pause and reflect on our journey. Much like the satisfaction one feels after a day spent exploring a city's nooks and crannies, understanding the nuances of our food choices gives us a sense of accomplishment.

Dr. Nowzaradan's guidance serves as a compass in our culinary adventures, helping us distinguish between the foods that fuel our journey and those that might lead us astray. Remember, every city, no matter how enchanting, has its pitfalls. But with caution and awareness, we can bypass these obstacles and keep our journey smooth.

Like any seasoned traveler, the key is in preparation. When we prepare for the challenges, when we arm ourselves with knowledge and a sense of purpose, the journey becomes a joy. The noisy streets of temptation become less daunting, and the allure of the unhealthy fades away, making room for choices that resonate with our health goals.

In the grand tapestry of life, every meal, every snack, is a thread. And with each healthy choice, we're weaving a narrative of vitality, longevity, and well-being. As you step out, map in hand, ready to navigate the bustling streets of life's dietary choices, remember: the journey is as significant as the destination. Savor each moment, each decision, and let the path you tread be one of vibrancy, health, and joy.

Chapter 5. Recipes for a Typical Week

Intro

Embarking on a weight loss journey often feels like navigating uncharted waters. With an abundance of dietary fads and conflicting advice available, it can be challenging to discern what truly works. Amidst this maze of information, Dr. Nowzaradan's diet philosophy emerges as a beacon of clarity. Rooted in decades of medical expertise and countless success stories, Dr. Now's approach is not just about shedding pounds but about adopting a holistic and sustainable lifestyle change. Welcome to Chapter 5, where we delve into an array of recipes designed to set beginners on a triumphant path without feeling overwhelmingly restrictive.

When we say "for beginners," we recognize the myriad challenges that newcomers often face when transitioning from their regular diets. It's crucial to acknowledge that any drastic change can be daunting, which is why these recipes have been crafted to be both appealing and in alignment with Dr. Now's principles without being too stringent. This gentle introduction ensures that one can ease into this new dietary regimen without feeling deprived, thus fostering a positive and enduring relationship with food.

Central to Dr. Nowzaradan's philosophy is the focus on high-protein meals. Proteins are the building blocks of our muscles and play a pivotal role in various bodily functions. A diet rich in protein not only aids muscle repair and growth but also helps in satiety, ensuring that hunger pangs are kept at bay. This is especially crucial for those embarking on their weight loss journeys, as it mitigates the urge to indulge in unhealthy snacking or overeating.

But why the emphasis on low fat and low carbs? Dietary fats, especially when consumed in large amounts from unhealthy sources, contribute significantly to weight gain and can lead to various health complications. Reducing fat intake, particularly from saturated and trans fats, promotes heart health and aids weight management. Similarly, while carbohydrates are essential as they provide our primary energy source, excessive consumption, especially of refined carbs, can result in weight gain and fluctuations in blood sugar levels. By moderating carb intake and choosing complex carbs over simple ones, you ensure a steady energy release, keeping you active and alert without unwanted weight gains.

The recipes curated in this chapter meticulously adhere to this triumvirate of high protein, low fat, and low carbs. They are not just nutritional powerhouses but are also palatable delights. From zesty shrimp skewers to heartwarming turkey-stuffed bell peppers, these recipes cater to varied taste buds while ensuring that you remain within the recommended caloric intake.

However, a note of caution: while these recipes are crafted following expert guidelines, individual dietary needs can vary. It's essential to adjust serving sizes and ingredient quantities to fit your unique nutritional requirements and caloric limits. Furthermore, before diving headfirst into any new diet or making significant changes to your existing one, it's always wise to consult with a nutritionist or a doctor. Personalized guidance can make the difference between a successful dietary transition and potential health complications.

As you flip through this chapter, remember that every meal, every ingredient, and every bite is a step towards a healthier, more vibrant you. With Dr. Nowzaradan's philosophy as your guide and these recipes as your toolkit, you are well-equipped to embark on a transformative journey towards better health and wellbeing.

Energizing Breakfasts

Recipe 1: Sunrise Spinach and Feta Omelette

- P.T.: 15 minutes
- Ingr.: 3 eggs, 1 cup fresh spinach, ¼ cup crumbled feta cheese, 1 tbsp olive oil, salt, and pepper.
- Serves: 1
- Mode of cooking: Stovetop
- Procedure: Heat olive oil in a non-stick pan. Sauté spinach until wilted. Beat the eggs, season with salt and   pepper, then pour over spinach. Once the omelette starts to set, sprinkle feta on one half, then fold. Serve hot.
- Nutritional values: 290 calories, 20g protein, 22g fat, 3g carbs.

Recipe 2: Almond Joy Overnight Oats

- P.T.: 10 minutes (plus overnight soaking)
- Ingr.: ½ cup rolled oats, 1 cup almond milk, 1 tbsp honey, 2 tbsp shredded coconut, 1 tbsp cocoa powder, 1 tbsp almond butter.
- Serves: 1
- Mode of cooking: No cook, refrigeration
- Procedure: Mix all ingredients in a jar. Refrigerate overnight. In the morning, give it a good stir and enjoy   cold or warmed up.
- Nutritional values: 370 calories, 9g protein, 18g fat, 49g carbs.

Recipe 3: Protein-Packed Banana Pancakes

- P.T.: 20 minutes
- Ingr.: 2 ripe bananas, 2 eggs, ¼ cup protein powder, ½ tsp baking powder, 1 tsp vanilla extract.
- Serves: 2
- Mode of cooking: Stovetop

- Procedure: Mash bananas. Mix in eggs, protein powder, baking powder, and vanilla. Cook in a non-stick pan like traditional pancakes. Serve with fresh fruit or a drizzle of honey.
- Nutritional values: 280 calories, 20g protein, 6g fat, 45g carbs.

Recipe 4: Nutty Chia Seed Pudding

- P.T.: 10 minutes (plus overnight soaking)
- Ingr.: 2 tbsp chia seeds, 1 cup almond milk, 1 tbsp honey, 1 tsp vanilla extract, 2 tbsp slivered almonds.
- Serves: 1
- Mode of cooking: No cook, refrigeration
- Procedure: Mix chia seeds, almond milk, honey, and vanilla in a jar. Refrigerate overnight. Top with almonds before serving.
- Nutritional values: 220 calories, 8g protein, 14g fat, 23g carbs.

Recipe 5: Zesty Avocado Toast

- P.T.: 10 minutes
- Ingr.: 1 slice whole-grain bread, ½ ripe avocado, 1 tsp lemon juice, chili flakes, salt, and pepper.
- Serves: 1
- Mode of cooking: Toaster
- Procedure: Toast bread. Mash avocado with lemon juice, salt, and chili flakes. Spread on toast.
- Nutritional values: 210 calories, 6g protein, 15g fat, 22g carbs.

Recipe 6: Refreshing Berry Smoothie

- P.T.: 5 minutes
- Ingr.: ½ cup strawberries, ½ cup blueberries, 1 cup Greek yogurt, 1 tbsp honey.
- Serves: 1
- Mode of cooking: Blender
- Procedure: Blend all ingredients until smooth. Pour into a glass and enjoy.

- Nutritional values: 250 calories, 15g protein, 2g fat, 50g carbs.

Recipe 7: Savory Veggie Muffins

- P.T.: 35 minutes

- Ingr.: 1 cup mixed veggies (e.g., zucchini, bell pepper), 2 eggs, ½ cup whole wheat flour, ¼ cup milk, 1 tsp baking powder, salt, and pepper.

- Serves: 6

- Mode of cookin: Baking

- Procedure: Mix all ingredients. Pour into muffin tins. Bake at 350°F for 25 minutes.

- Nutritional values: 80 calories, 5g protein, 2g fat, 12g carbs.

Recipe 8: Whole Grain Waffles with Blueberry Compote

- P.T.: 30 minutes

-Ingr.: Whole grain waffle mix, Blueberries, Honey.

- Serves: 2 waffles

-Mode of cooking: Baking & Simmering

- Procedure: Prepare waffles. Cook blueberries with honey for compote. Pour over waffles.

- Nutritional values: Approx. 290 calories, 6g protein, 8g fat, 50g carbs.

Recipe 9: Smoked Salmon Bagel

- P.T.: 15 minutes

- Ingr.: 1 whole grain bagel, 2 tbsp cream cheese, 3 slices smoked salmon, 1 tsp capers, 1 slice red onion, 1 tsp fresh dill.

- Serves: 1

- Mode of cooking: Assembly

- Procedure: Toast bagel. Spread cream cheese. Top with salmon, capers, onion, and dill.

- Nutritional values: 350 calories, 25g protein, 15g fat, 32g carbs.

Recipe 10: Fruity Quinoa Bowl

- P.T.: 25 minutes

- Ingr.: ½ cup quinoa, 1 cup water, ½ cup mixed berries, 1 tbsp honey, 2 tbsp chopped nuts.

- Serves: 1

- Mode of cooking: Stovetop

- Procedure: Cook quinoa. Let cool. Mix with berries, honey, and nuts.

- Nutritional values: 310 calories, 9g protein, 10g fat, 49g carbs.

Recipe 11: Mediterranean Breakfast Wrap

- P.T.: 20 minutes

- Ingr.: 1 whole grain tortilla, 2 eggs, ¼ cup chopped tomatoes, ¼ cup chopped cucumbers, ¼ cup crumbled feta cheese, 1 tbsp tzatziki sauce, 1 tbsp chopped olives.

- Serves: 1

- Mode of cooking: Stovetop

- Procedure: Scramble eggs in a non-stick pan. Warm the tortilla. Place scrambled eggs, tomatoes, cucumbers, feta, and olives in the center. Drizzle with tzatziki. Roll up and enjoy.

- Nutritional values: 400 calories, 20g protein, 18g fat, 42g carbs.

Recipe 12: Mango Tango Smoothie Bowl

- P.T.: 10 minutes

- Ingr.: 1 ripe mango, ½ cup Greek yogurt, ½ cup almond milk, 1 tbsp chia seeds, 1 tbsp shredded coconut, 2 tbsp granola.

- Serves: 1

- Mode of cooking: Blender

- Procedure: Blend mango, yogurt, and almond milk until smooth. Pour into a bowl. Top with chia seeds, coconut, and granola.

- Nutritional values: 360 calories, 12g protein, 10g fat, 58g carbs.

Recipe 13: Sweet Potato Hash with Poached Eggs

- P.T.: 35 minutes

- Ingr.: 1 medium sweet potato, diced, 1 small red onion, chopped, 1 bell pepper, chopped, 2 eggs, 1 tbsp olive oil, salt, and pepper.

- Serves: 2

- Mode of cooking: Stovetop

- Procedure: Sauté sweet potato, onion, and bell pepper in olive oil until tender. In a separate pan, poach eggs. Serve hash with poached eggs on top.

- Nutritional values: 280 calories, 10g protein, 12g fat, 35g carbs.

Recipe 14: Wholesome Grain and Fruit Parfait

- P.T.: 15 minutes

- Ingr.: ½ cup cooked quinoa, ½ cup Greek yogurt, ½ cup mixed berries, 1 tbsp honey, 1 tbsp slivered almonds, 1 tbsp sunflower seeds.

- Serves: 1

- Mode of cooking: Layering

- Procedure: Layer quinoa, yogurt, and berries in a tall glass or jar. Drizzle with honey. Top with almonds and sunflower seeds.

- Nutritional values: 340 calories, 14g protein, 10g fat, 53g carbs.

Recipe 15: Nut and Seed Protein Bars

- P.T.: 40 minutes (plus cooling time)

- Ingr.: 1 cup rolled oats, ½ cup protein powder, ½ cup almond butter, ¼ cup honey, ¼ cup mixed nuts (almonds, walnuts), 2 tbsp chia seeds, 2 tbsp flax seeds, 2 tbsp pumpkin seeds.

- Serves: 8

- Mode of cooking: Baking

- Procedure: Mix all ingredients in a bowl. Press mixture into a lined baking dish. Bake at 350°F for 25 minutes. Cool and cut into bars.

- Nutritional values: 260 calories, 14g protein, 15g fat, 25g carbs.

Recipe 16: Creamy Avocado Toast with Poached Eggs

- P.T.: 15 minutes

- Ingr.: Whole grain toast, 1 ripe avocado, chili flakes (optional), sea salt, lemon (optional), 1 egg.

- Serves: 1

- Mode of cooking: Toasting & Poaching

- Procedure: Toast bread to desired crispness. Slice avocado and layer onto toast. Sprinkle with chili flakes, sea salt, and a dash of lemon. Poach egg and place atop the avocado.

- Nutritional values: Approx. 350 calories, 12g protein, 25g fat, 25g carbs.

Recipe 17: Greek Yogurt Parfait with Mixed Berries and Granola

- P.T.: 10 minutes

- Ingr.: Greek yogurt, Mixed berries, Granola.

- Serves: 1

- Mode of cooking: Layering

- Procedure: In a glass, layer yogurt, berries, and granola. Repeat until satisfied.

- Nutritional values: Approx. 250 calories, 15g protein, 3g fat, 40g carbs.

Recipe 18: Tropical Smoothie Bowl

- P.T.: 10 minutes

- Ingr.: Mangoes, Bananas, Pineapples, Almond milk, Chia seeds, Coconut flakes, Kiwi.

- Serves: 1

- Mode of cooking: Blending

- Procedure: Blend fruits with almond milk. Pour into bowl, top with chia, coconut, and kiwi.

- Nutritional values: Approx. 330 calories, 6g protein, 10g fat, 58g carbs.

Recipe 19: Quinoa Porridge with Cinnamon and Apple

- P.T.: 20 minutes

- Ingr: Quinoa, Almond milk, Apples, Cinnamon, Honey (optional).

- Serves: 1

- Mode of cooking: Boiling

- Procedure: Cook quinoa in milk, add apples and cinnamon. Sweeten with honey.

- Nutritional values: Approx. 250 calories, 8g protein, 3g fat, 50g carbs.

Recipe 20: Banana and Walnut Muffins

- P.T.: 40 minutes

- Ingr.: Bananas, Chopped walnuts, Standard muffin ingredients.

- Serves: 12 muffins

- Mode of cooking: Baking

- Procedure: Create muffin batter with bananas, add walnuts. Bake.

- Nutritional values: Approx. 190 calories, 4g protein, 8g fat, 27g carbs.

Balanced lunches

Recipe 1: Mediterranean Quinoa Salad

- P.T.: 30 minutes

- Ingr.:

  - 1 cup quinoa

  - 2 cups water

  - 1 cup diced cucumber

  - 1 cup cherry tomatoes, halved

  - 1/2 cup diced red onion

  - 1/2 cup feta cheese

  - 2 tbsp olive oil

  - 1 tbsp lemon juice

  - Salt and pepper to taste

  - 1/4 cup chopped parsley

- Serves: 4

- Mode of cooking: Stovetop

- Procedure:

1. Rinse the quinoa thoroughly. In a pot, bring 2 cups of water to a boil. Add quinoa, reduce heat, cover, and simmer for 15 minutes or until water is absorbed. Allow it to cool.

2. In a large bowl, mix quinoa, cucumber, cherry tomatoes, red onion, and feta cheese.

3. In a small bowl, whisk together olive oil, lemon juice, salt, and pepper. Pour dressing over quinoa mixture.

4. Garnish with parsley before serving.

- Nutritional values: Approximately 250 calories, 8g protein, 12g fat, 30g carbs.

Recipe 2: Thai Basil Chicken

- P.T.: 20 minutes

- Ingr.:

  - 400g chicken breast, thinly sliced

  - 2 tbsp olive oil

  - 3 garlic cloves, minced

  - 2 Thai chilies, finely chopped

  - 1 red bell pepper, sliced

  - 1/2 cup green beans, chopped

  - 2 tbsp low-sodium soy sauce

  - 1 tbsp fish sauce

  - 1 tsp sugar substitute

  - 1/2 cup fresh basil leaves

- Serves: 4

- Mode of cooking: Stovetop

- Procedure:

1. In a wok or large pan, heat the olive oil over medium heat. Add garlic and chilies and sauté for 1 minute.

2. Add chicken slices and cook until browned.

3. Add red bell pepper and green beans, sauté for another 3-4 minutes.

4. In a bowl, mix together soy sauce, fish sauce, and sugar substitute. Pour this over the chicken.

5. Stir in fresh basil leaves and cook for another minute. Serve hot.

- Nutritional values: Approximately 200 calories, 25g protein, 8g fat, 5g carbs.

Recipe 3: Spinach and Mushroom Frittata

- P.T.: 25 minutes
- Ingr.:
  - 6 large eggs
  - 1/4 cup milk
  - Salt and pepper to taste
  - 1 tbsp olive oil
  - 1 onion, diced
  - 2 cups baby spinach
  - 1 cup mushrooms, sliced
  - 1/4 cup grated parmesan cheese
- Serves: 4
- Mode of cooking: Oven
- Procedure:

1. Preheat oven to 400°F (200°C).

2. In a bowl, whisk together eggs, milk, salt, and pepper.

3. In an ovenproof skillet, heat olive oil over medium heat. Add onions and sauté until translucent. Add mushrooms and cook for 5 minutes.

4. Add spinach and cook until wilted.

5. Pour egg mixture over vegetables in the skillet and sprinkle with parmesan cheese.

6. Transfer skillet to oven and bake for 10-12 minutes or until frittata is set.

- Nutritional values: Approximately 180 calories, 12g protein, 12g fat, 4g carbs.

Recipe 4: Moroccan Lentil Soup

- P.T.: 40 minutes
- Ingr.:
  - 1 cup lentils, rinsed
  - 1 tbsp olive oil
  - 1 onion, diced
  - 2 garlic cloves, minced
  - 2 carrots, diced
  - 2 celery stalks, diced
  - 1 tsp ground cumin
  - 1/2 tsp paprika
  - 4 cups low-sodium vegetable broth
  - Salt and pepper to taste
  - 2 tbsp chopped cilantro for garnish
- Serves: 4
- Mode of cooking: Stovetop
- Procedure:

  1. In a pot, heat olive oil over medium heat. Add onions, garlic, carrots, and celery. Sauté for 5 minutes.

  2. Add cumin, paprika, lentils, and vegetable broth. Bring to a boil.

  3. Reduce heat, cover, and simmer for 30 minutes or until lentils are tender.

  4. Season with salt and pepper. Garnish with cilantro before serving.

- Nutritional values: Approximately 200 calories, 12g protein, 3g fat, 35g carbs.

Recipe 5: Mexican Grilled Chicken Salad

- P.T.: 30 minutes
- Ingr.:
  - 2 chicken breasts
  - 1 tbsp olive oil
  - 1 tsp cumin
  - 1 tsp paprika

- 1 tsp garlic powder

- Salt and pepper to taste

- 4 cups mixed salad greens

- 1/2 cup black beans, rinsed and drained

- 1/4 cup corn kernels

- 1/2 avocado, sliced

- 1/4 cup salsa for dressing

- Serves: 4

- Mode of cooking: Grill

- Procedure:

1. Mix olive oil, cumin, paprika, garlic powder, salt, and pepper in a bowl. Marinate chicken breasts in this mixture for at least 15 minutes.

2. Preheat grill over medium heat. Grill chicken for 6-7 minutes on each side or until cooked through. Let it rest for a few minutes and then slice.

3. On a serving plate, lay out salad greens. Top with black beans, corn, avocado slices, and grilled chicken.

4. Drizzle salsa over the salad before serving.

- Nutritional values: Approximately 250 calories, 30g protein, 9g fat, 10g carbs.

Recipe 6: Indian Spiced Chickpea Salad

- P.T.: 20 minutes

- Ingr.:

- 1 can (400g) chickpeas, rinsed and drained

- 1 cucumber, diced

- 1 tomato, diced

- 1/4 cup red onion, finely chopped

- 1 green chili, finely chopped (optional)

- 2 tbsp fresh cilantro, chopped

- 1 tbsp fresh lemon juice

- 1/2 tsp ground cumin

- Salt to taste

- Serves: 4

- Mode of cooking: No cooking required

- Procedure:

   1. In a large bowl, combine chickpeas, cucumber, tomato, red onion, and green chili.

   2. In a small bowl, mix lemon juice, cumin, and salt. Pour over the chickpea mixture.

   3. Toss to combine and garnish with fresh cilantro before serving.

- Nutritional values: Approximately 200 calories, 8g protein, 3g fat, 35g carbs.

Recipe 7: Japanese Miso Soup with Tofu

- P.T.: 20 minutes

- Ingr.:

   - 4 cups water

   - 2 tbsp miso paste

   - 1/2 cup diced tofu

   - 2 green onions, sliced

   - 1 sheet nori seaweed, torn into pieces

   - 1/2 cup spinach leaves

- Serves: 4

- Mode of cooking: Stovetop

- Procedure:

   1. In a pot, bring water to a boil. Lower the heat and dissolve miso paste in the water using a whisk.

   2. Add tofu, green onions, and nori to the pot. Simmer for 5 minutes.

   3. Add spinach and cook for another 2 minutes. Serve hot.

- Nutritional values: Approximately 60 calories, 4g protein, 2g fat, 5g carbs.

Recipe 8: Italian Zucchini Noodles with Pesto

- P.T.: 15 minutes
- Ingr.:
  - 2 large zucchinis, spiralized
  - 2 tbsp pesto sauce (store-bought or homemade with basil, garlic, pine nuts, parmesan, olive oil, salt)
  - 1/4 cup cherry tomatoes, halved
  - 2 tbsp grated parmesan cheese
  - Salt and pepper to taste
- Serves: 2
- Mode of cooking: Stovetop
- Procedure:
  1. In a pan, heat a tablespoon of olive oil and sauté the spiralized zucchini for 3-4 minutes.
  2. Add pesto sauce, cherry tomatoes, salt, and pepper. Mix well.
  3. Serve hot, garnished with grated parmesan cheese.
- Nutritional values: Approximately 150 calories, 5g protein, 11g fat, 10g carbs.

Recipe 9: French Ratatouille

- P.T.: 45 minutes
- Ingr.:
  - 1 eggplant, diced
  - 1 zucchini, diced
  - 1 red bell pepper, diced
  - 1 onion, chopped
  - 2 garlic cloves, minced
  - 1 can (400g) diced tomatoes
  - 2 tbsp olive oil
  - 1/2 tsp dried thyme
  - Salt and pepper to taste

- Fresh basil for garnish

- Serves: 4

- Mode of cooking: Stovetop

- Procedure:

    1. In a large pan, heat olive oil. Add onions and garlic and sauté until translucent.

    2. Add eggplant, zucchini, and bell pepper. Cook for about 10 minutes.

    3. Add tomatoes, thyme, salt, and pepper. Cover and simmer for 30 minutes.

    4. Garnish with fresh basil before serving.

- Nutritional values: Approximately 120 calories, 3g protein, 7g fat, 15g carbs.

Recipe 10: Grilled lean beef with Salad

- P.T.: 30 minutes

- Ingr.:

    - 400g lean beef steaks

    - Salt and pepper to taste

    - 1 tbsp olive oil

    - 4 cups mixed salad greens

    - 1/4 cup cherry tomatoes, halved

    - 1/4 cup sliced cucumber

    - 1/4 cup diced red onion

    - 1 tbsp balsamic vinegar

- Serves: 4

- Mode of cooking: Grill

- Procedure:

    1. Season the lean beef steaks with salt and pepper.

    2. Preheat grill over medium heat. Drizzle olive oil on the steaks and grill for about 3-4 minutes on each side or until cooked to desired doneness.

    3. In a bowl, combine salad greens, cherry tomatoes, cucumber, and red onion.

    4. Slice the grilled lean beef and place it on top of the salad. Drizzle with balsamic vinegar before serving.

- Nutritional values: Approximately 200 calories, 25g protein, 9g fat, 5g carbs.

Recipe 11: Japanese Sushi (Maki)

- P.T.: 45 minutes
- Ingredients:
  - 2 cups sushi rice
  - 2.5 cups water
  - 1/3 cup rice vinegar
  - 3 tbsp sugar
  - 1 tsp salt
  - Nori seaweed sheets
  - Choice of raw fish (e.g. salmon, tuna)
  - Choice of vegetables (e.g. cucumber, avocado)
  - Soy sauce for serving
- Servings: 4
- Cooking method: Stovetop and sushi rolling mat
- Instructions:
  1. Rinse the rice until the water runs clear. Cook the rice with 2.5 cups of water.
  2. Once cooked, let it cool slightly. Mix the rice vinegar, sugar, and salt, then pour over the rice. Gently mix.
  3. On a sushi rolling mat, lay out a nori sheet. Spread a thin layer of rice, leaving a space at the edge of the nori.
  4. Add strips of fish and vegetables in the center.
  5. Gently roll using the mat.
  6. Slice into bite-sized pieces and serve with soy sauce.
- Nutritional Values: Approx. 300 calories, 10g protein, 1g fats, 65g carbohydrates.

Recipe 12: Moroccan Lentil Soup

- P.T.: 45 minutes
- Ingr.:
  - 1 cup dried lentils, rinsed
  - 1 onion, chopped
  - 2 garlic cloves, minced

- 1 carrot, diced

- 1 celery stalk, diced

- 1 can (400g) diced tomatoes

- 6 cups vegetable broth

- 1 tsp ground cumin

- 1/2 tsp ground turmeric

- 1/2 tsp paprika

- Salt and pepper to taste

- 2 tbsp fresh cilantro, chopped

- Serves: 6

- Mode of cooking: Stovetop

- Procedure:

1. In a large pot, heat a tablespoon of olive oil. Sauté onions and garlic until translucent.

2. Add carrots and celery and cook for 5 minutes.

3. Add lentils, tomatoes, vegetable broth, cumin, turmeric, paprika, salt, and pepper.

4. Bring to a boil, then reduce heat and simmer for 30-35 minutes until lentils are soft.

5. Garnish with fresh cilantro before serving.

- Nutritional values: Approximately 150 calories, 9g protein, 0.5g fat, 28g carbs.

Recipe 13: Greek Tzatziki Dip

- P.T.: 10 minutes

- Ingr.:

- 1 cup Greek yogurt

- 1 cucumber, finely grated and drained

- 2 garlic cloves, minced

- 1 tbsp fresh dill, chopped

- 1 tbsp fresh lemon juice

- Salt and pepper to taste

- 1 tbsp olive oil

- Serves: 4

- Mode of cooking: Mixing bowl

- Procedure:

  1. In a bowl, combine Greek yogurt, grated cucumber, garlic, dill, and lemon juice. Mix well.

  2. Season with salt and pepper.

  3. Drizzle with olive oil before serving. Enjoy with fresh pita bread or vegetable sticks.

- Nutritional values: Approximately 80 calories, 5g protein, 4g fat, 5g carbs.

Recipe 14: South African Bobotie

- P.T.: 60 minutes

- Ingr.:

  - 500g lean ground beef

  - 1 onion, chopped

  - 2 garlic cloves, minced

  - 2 slices bread, soaked in milk

  - 2 tbsp curry powder

  - 1 apple, grated

  - 1/2 cup raisins

  - 2 eggs

  - 1 cup milk

  - Salt and pepper to taste

  - Bay leaves for garnish

- Serves: 6

- Mode of cooking: Oven

- Procedure:

  1. Preheat oven to 180°C (350°F).

  2. In a pan, sauté onion and garlic until translucent. Add ground beef and cook until browned.

3. Add curry powder, grated apple, and raisins. Season with salt and pepper.

4. Squeeze out excess milk from the bread and mix it into the meat mixture.

5. Transfer the mixture to an ovenproof dish.

6. In a separate bowl, whisk together eggs and milk. Pour over the meat mixture.

7. Place bay leaves on top.

8. Bake for 30-35 minutes until the top is golden.

- Nutritional values: Approximately 320 calories, 25g protein, 15g fat, 20g carbs.

Recipe 15: Spanish Gazpacho

- P.T.: 15 minutes (+ chilling time)

- Ingr.:

  - 6 ripe tomatoes, chopped

  - 1 cucumber, peeled and chopped

  - 1 bell pepper, chopped

  - 1 small red onion, chopped

  - 2 garlic cloves

  - 3 cups tomato juice

  - 1/4 cup red wine vinegar

  - 1/4 cup olive oil

  - Salt and pepper to taste

- Serves: 6

- Mode of cooking: Blender

- Procedure:

1. In a blender, combine tomatoes, cucumber, bell pepper, onion, and garlic. Blend until smooth.

2. Add tomato juice, red wine vinegar, olive oil, salt, and pepper. Blend again to combine.

3. Chill in the refrigerator for at least 2 hours before serving.

- Nutritional values: Approximately 120 calories, 2g protein, 7g fat, 15g carbs.

Recipe 16: Zucchini Noodle Stir-Fry

- P.T.: 20 minutes

- Ingredients:

  - 2 large zucchinis, spiralized

  - 1 bell pepper, thinly sliced

  - 1 carrot, julienned

  - 2 green onions, chopped

  - 1 garlic clove, minced

  - 2 tbsp soy sauce

  - 1 tbsp olive oil

  - 1 tsp sesame seeds (optional)

- Servings: 2

- Cooking method: Stovetop

- Instructions:

  1. Heat olive oil in a large skillet over medium heat.

  2. Add garlic and sauté until fragrant.

  3. Add bell pepper and carrot, cooking until slightly softened.

  4. Stir in zucchini noodles and cook for an additional 2 minutes.

  5. Pour in soy sauce and toss to combine.

  6. Serve hot, garnished with green onions and sesame seeds.

- Nutritional Values: Approx. 120 calories, 3g protein, 7g fats, 10g carbohydrates.

Recipe 17: Spiced Grilled Chicken Salad

- P.T.: 25 minutes

-Ingredients:

  - 2 boneless chicken breasts

  - 1 tsp paprika

  - 1 tsp garlic powder

  - Salt and pepper, to taste

  - 2 cups mixed salad greens (e.g. arugula, spinach, romaine)

  - 1/4 red onion, thinly sliced

- 10 cherry tomatoes, halved

- 1 tbsp olive oil

- 1 tbsp balsamic vinegar

- Servings: 2

- Cooking metho: Grilling

- Instructions:

1. Preheat the grill to medium-high.

2. Season chicken breasts with paprika, garlic powder, salt, and pepper.

3. Grill chicken for 6-7 minutes on each side or until cooked through.

4. Let the chicken rest for a few minutes, then slice.

5. In a large bowl, combine salad greens, red onion, and cherry tomatoes.

6. In a separate bowl, whisk together olive oil and balsamic vinegar.

7. Toss the salad with the dressing and top with sliced chicken.

- Nutritional Values: Approx. 230 calories, 28g protein, 10g fats, 5g carbohydrates.

Recipe 18: Cauliflower Risotto

- P.T.: 30 minutes

- Ingredients:

- 1 large cauliflower head, riced in a food processor

- 1 small onion, diced

- 1 garlic clove, minced

- 1 cup chicken or vegetable broth

- 1/4 cup grated Parmesan cheese

- 2 tbsp olive oil

- Fresh parsley, chopped, for garnish

- Salt and pepper, to taste

- Servings: 4

- Cooking method: Stovetop

- Instructions:

1. Heat olive oil in a large skillet over medium heat.

2. Add onion and sauté until translucent.

3. Stir in minced garlic and cook for an additional minute.

4. Add riced cauliflower to the skillet, stirring occasionally for about 5 minutes.

5. Gradually pour in broth and cook, stirring occasionally until the cauliflower is tender.

6. Stir in Parmesan cheese, season with salt and pepper.

7. Serve hot, garnished with fresh parsley.

- Nutritional Values: Approx. 150 calories, 6g protein, 10g fats, 10g carbohydrates.

Recipe 19: Indian Chicken Curry

- P.T.: 40 minutes

- Ingredients:

  - 17.5 oz chicken breast, cubed

  - 1 onion, chopped

  - 2 garlic cloves, minced

  - 0.8-inch ginger piece, grated

  - 2 tbsp curry paste

  - 13.5 fl oz coconut milk

  - 1 tbsp oil

  - Salt, to taste

  - Fresh cilantro for garnish

- Servings: 4

- Cooking method: Stovetop

- Instructions:

  1. In a pot, heat the oil and sauté the onion until translucent.

  2. Add the garlic and ginger and cook for another 2 minutes.

  3. Stir in the curry paste.

  4. Add the chicken and cook until uniformly browned.

  5. Pour in the coconut milk and bring to a boil. Reduce the heat and simmer for 20 minutes.

  6. Garnish with fresh cilantro before serving.

- Nutritional Values: Approx. 350 calories, 30g protein, 20g fats, 10g carbohydrates.

Recipe 20: Mexican Tamales

- P.T.: 3 hours

- Ingredients:

  - 2 cups masa harina (corn flour)

  - 1 tsp baking powder

  - 1/2 tsp salt

  - 1/2 cup lard

  - 1.5 cups chicken broth

  - Corn husks, soaked in water

  - Choice of filling (chicken, pork, peppers, cheese)

- Servings: 6

- Cooking method: Steaming

- Instructions:

  1. In a large bowl, combine the masa harina, baking powder, and salt. Add the lard and mix until crumbly.

  2. Gradually add the chicken broth, mixing until a dough forms.

  3. Spread a portion of the dough in the center of a corn husk.

  4. Place your choice of filling in the center.

  5. Fold the sides of the husk over the filling, then fold the ends to seal.

  6. Steam the tamales for 2-3 hours.

  7. Serve hot.

- Nutritional Values: Approx. 250 calories, 7g protein, 12g fats, 30g carbohydrates.

Healthy snacks

Recipe 1: Cucumber & Herb Cottage Cheese Boats

- P.T.: 10 minutes
- Ingr.:
  - 1 large cucumber, halved and seeds removed
  - 1/2 cup non-fat cottage cheese
  - 1 tbsp fresh chives, finely chopped
  - 1 tbsp fresh parsley, finely chopped
  - Salt and pepper to taste
  - Paprika for garnish (optional)
- Serves: 2
- Mode of cooking: No-cook
- Procedure:

  1. In a small bowl, mix together the cottage cheese, chives, parsley, salt, and pepper.

  2. Scoop the mixture into the hollowed center of the cucumber halves.

  3. Sprinkle with paprika, if using, for an extra touch of color and flavor.

  4. Slice into bite-sized pieces and serve immediately.
- Nutritional Values: Approx. 40 calories, 7g protein, 0g fat, 3g carbohydrates.

Recipe 2: Spiced Turkey Jerky

- P.T.: 24 hours (includes marination)
- Ingr.:
  - 200g turkey breast, thinly sliced
  - 1 tsp smoked paprika
  - 1/2 tsp garlic powder
  - 1/2 tsp onion powder
  - Salt to taste
- Serves: 4
- Mode of cooking: Oven-dried

- Procedure:

    1. Combine all spices and rub them on turkey slices.

    2. Lay turkey slices on a baking tray.

    3. Dry in an oven at the lowest setting for 4-6 hours or until jerky-like consistency.

    4. Store in a cool, dry place.

- Nutritional Values: Approx. 70 calories, 14g protein, 1g fat, 1g carbohydrates.

Recipe 3: Boiled Egg with Bresaola

-P.T.: 10 minutes

- Ingr.:

    - 1 boiled eggs

    - 50g bresaola

- Serves: 2

- Mode of cooking: Boiling

- Procedure:

    1. Boil eggs to desired hardness.

    2. Peel and serve with slices of bresaola.

- Nutritional Values: Approx. 70 calories, 10g protein, 2,5g fat, 0,5g carbohydrates.

Recipe 4: Veggie Sticks with Hummus

- P.T.: 10 minutes

- Ingr.:

    - 2 celery stalks, chopped

    - 1 carrot, sliced

    - 100g hummus

- Serves: 2

- Mode of cooking: No-cook

- Procedure:

    1. Clean and chop the veggies.

    2. Serve with hummus for dipping.

-Nutritional Values: Approx. 90 calories, 3g protein, 5g fat, 8g carbohydrates.

Recipe 5: Almond & Blueberry Protein Bites

- P.T.: 15 minutes
- Ingr.:
  - 100g almonds, crushed
  - 50g blueberries
  - 2 tbsp Greek yogurt
- Serves: 4
- Mode of cooking: No-cook
- Procedure:
  1. Mix all ingredients in a bowl.
  2. Roll into bite-sized balls and refrigerate for 1 hour before serving.
- Nutritional Values: Approx. 90 calories, 4g protein, 7g fat, 4g carbohydrates.

Recipe 6: Spinach and Feta Stuffed Mushrooms

- P.T.: 20 minutes
- Ingr.:
  - 6 large mushrooms, stems removed
  - 100g spinach, chopped
  - 50g feta cheese, crumbled
  - 1 tsp olive oil
  - Salt and pepper to taste
- Serves: 3
- Mode of cooking: Baking
- Procedure:
  1. Preheat oven to 350°F (175°C).
  2. In a pan, heat olive oil and sauté spinach until wilted.
  3. Mix in crumbled feta, salt, and pepper.
  4. Stuff each mushroom cap with the spinach-feta mixture.
  5. Place on a baking sheet and bake for 15 minutes or until mushrooms are tender.
- Nutritional Values: Approx. 70 calories, 5g protein, 4g fat, 3g carbohydrates.

Recipe 7: Zucchini Chips

- P.T.: 2 hours 10 minutes

- Ingr.:

  - 1 zucchini, thinly sliced

  - 1 tsp olive oil

  - Salt and pepper to taste

- Serves: 2

- Mode of cooking: Baking

- Procedure:

  1. Preheat oven to 225°F (105°C).

  2. Toss zucchini slices in olive oil, salt, and pepper.

  3. Lay slices on a baking sheet in a single layer.

  4. Bake for 2 hours, turning halfway through until crisp.

- Nutritional Values: Approx. 45 calories, 1g protein, 3g fat, 4g carbohydrates.

Recipe 8: Zucchini Rolls with Tuna Filling

- P.T.: 15 minutes

- Ingr.:

  - 1 medium zucchini, sliced into thin long strips using a mandolin or vegetable peeler

  - 1 can (5 oz.) light tuna in water, drained

  - 2 tbsp non-fat Greek yogurt

  - 1 tbsp lemon juice

  - Salt and pepper to taste

  - Fresh dill for garnish (optional)

- Serves: 2 (around 3-4 rolls per serving)

- Mode of cooking: No-cook

- Procedure:

  1. In a bowl, mix together the drained tuna, Greek yogurt, and lemon juice. Season with salt and pepper to taste.

  2. Lay out the zucchini strips flat on a clean surface.

3. Place a small amount of the tuna mixture on one end of each zucchini strip.

4. Roll the zucchini strip to encase the tuna mixture.

5. Garnish with dill, if desired.

6. Serve immediately or refrigerate for later.

- Nutritional Values: Approx. 40 calories, 8g protein, 0.5g fat, 2g carbohydrates.

Recipe 9: Broccoli & Cauliflower Bites

- P.T.: 25 minutes

- Ingr.:

  - 1 cup broccoli florets, steamed and finely chopped

  - 1 cup cauliflower florets, steamed and finely chopped

  - 1 garlic clove, minced

  - 2 tbsp egg whites

  - Salt and pepper to taste

- Serves: 2 (around 5-6 bites per serving)

- Mode of cooking: Baking

- Procedure:

  1. Preheat oven to 400°F (200°C) and line a baking tray with parchment paper.

  2. In a mixing bowl, combine chopped broccoli, chopped cauliflower, minced garlic, and egg whites. Season with salt and pepper.

  3. Shape the mixture into small bite-sized balls and place them on the prepared baking tray.

  4. Bake in the preheated oven for 15-20 minutes or until they are golden brown and firm.

  5. Let cool slightly before serving.

- Nutritional Values: Approx. 30 calories, 3g protein, 0.5g fat, 4g carbohydrates.

Recipe 10: Grilled Asparagus Spears

- P.T.: 15 minutes

- Ingr.:

  - 12 asparagus spears, trimmed

  - 1 tsp olive oil

  - Salt and pepper to taste

- Serves: 2

- Mode of cooking: Grilling

- Procedure:

  1. Preheat grill to medium-high heat.

  2. Toss asparagus in olive oil, salt, and pepper.

  3. Grill for 7-10 minutes, turning occasionally until tender and slightly charred.

- Nutritional Values: Approx. 40 calories, 2g protein, 2.5g fat, 4g carbohydrates.

Recipe 11: Spinach & Mushroom Stuffed Bell Peppers

- P.T.: 25 minutes

- Ingr.:

  - 2 large bell peppers (any color), halved and seeds removed

  - 1 cup fresh spinach, chopped

  - 1/2 cup mushrooms, finely chopped

  - 1 garlic clove, minced

  - Salt and pepper to taste

  - 2 tbsp water

- Serves: 2 (1 bell pepper each)

- Mode of cooking: Saute and bake

- Procedure:

  1. Preheat oven to 375°F (190°C).

  2. In a non-stick pan over medium heat, sauté mushrooms and garlic in 2 tbsp of water until mushrooms are tender, about 3-4 minutes. Add the chopped spinach and cook until wilted.

  3. Season the mixture with salt and pepper.

4. Stuff each bell pepper half with the spinach and mushroom mixture.

5. Place the stuffed bell peppers on a baking tray and bake for 15-20 minutes or until the peppers are tender.

6. Remove from oven and serve immediately.

- Nutritional Values: Approx. 45 calories, 2g protein, 0g fat, 10g carbohydrates.

Recipe 12: Cucumber Hummus Bites

- P.T.: 15 minutes
- Ingr.:
  - 1 cucumber, sliced into rounds
- 100g hummus
- Paprika for garnish
- Serves: 4
- Mode of cooking: No-cook
- Procedure:

   1. Spread a small amount of hummus onto each cucumber slice.

   2. Garnish with a sprinkle of paprika.

   3. Chill before serving.

- Nutritional Values: Approx. 50 calories, 2g protein, 2g fat, 4g carbohydrates.

Recipe 13: Turkey Roll-Ups

- P.T.: 10 minutes
- Ingr.:
  - 4 turkey slices
  - 1/4 cup cream cheese (low-fat)
  - 1/4 bell pepper, thinly sliced
- Serves: 2
- Mode of cooking: No-cook
- Procedure:

   1. Lay turkey slices flat. Spread a thin layer of cream cheese over each slice.

   2. Place bell pepper slices at one end of the turkey slice.

3. Roll up tightly and cut into bite-sized pieces.

- Nutritional Values: Approx. 80 calories, 7g protein, 3g fat, 1g carbohydrates.

Recipe 14: Baked Kale Chips

- P.T.: 20 minutes
- Ingr.:
  - 2 cups kale, washed and torn into bite-sized pieces
  - 1 tsp olive oil
  - Salt and pepper to taste
- Serves: 2
- Mode of cooking: Baking
- Procedure:
  1. Preheat oven to 350°F (175°C).
  2. Mix kale with olive oil, salt, and pepper in a bowl.
  3. Spread on a baking sheet in a single layer.
  4. Bake for 10-15 minutes or until edges are brown but not burnt.
- Nutritional Values: Approx. 50 calories, 2g protein, 2.5g fat, 5g carbohydrates.

Recipe 15: Spinach & Tomato Stuffed Bell Peppers

- P.T.: 30 minutes
- Ingr.:
  - 2 large bell peppers (any color), halved and seeds removed
  - 1 cup fresh spinach, chopped
  - 1 medium tomato, finely diced
  - Salt and pepper to taste
  - 1 tsp olive oil
- Serves: 2 (1 half pepper per serving)
- Mode of cooking: Baking
- Procedure:
  1. Preheat oven to 375°F (190°C).

2. In a bowl, mix the chopped spinach and diced tomato. Season with a pinch of salt and pepper.

3. Brush the outside of the bell peppers lightly with olive oil.

4. Stuff each bell pepper half with the spinach and tomato mixture.

5. Place the stuffed peppers on a baking tray and bake for 20-25 minutes, or until the peppers are soft.

6. Serve warm.

- Nutritional Values: Approx. 60 calories, 2g protein, 1g fat, 8g carbohydrates.

Recipe 16: Celery Peanut Butter Boats

- P.T.: 10 minutes

- Ingr.:

  - 4 celery sticks, washed and trimmed

  - 2 tbsp natural peanut butter (no sugar added)

  - Chia seeds for garnish (optional)

- Serves: 2 (2 sticks per serving)

- Mode of cooking: No-cook

- Procedure:

  1. Spread half a tablespoon of peanut butter into the groove of each celery stick.

  2. If desired, sprinkle with chia seeds for added texture and nutrition.

  3. Serve immediately.

- Nutritional Values: Approx. 50 calories, 2g protein, 3g fat, 2g carbohydrates.

Recipe 17: Cucumber Hummus Bites

- P.T.: 10 minutes

- Ingr.:

  - 1 large cucumber, sliced into rounds

  - 1/4 cup hummus (opt for a low-fat variant if available)

  - Fresh parsley for garnish

  - Paprika for sprinkling (optional)

- Serves: 4 (about 5-6 slices per serving)

- Mode of cooking: No-cook

- Procedure:

    1. Lay out cucumber slices on a plate.

    2. Dollop a small amount of hummus on each slice.

    3. Garnish with fresh parsley and a sprinkle of paprika if desired.

    4. Serve immediately.

- Nutritional Values: Approx. 30 calories, 1g protein, 1g fat, 3g carbohydrates.

Recipe 18: Spinach and Feta Stuffed Mushrooms

- P.T.: 30 minutes

- Ingr.:

    - 6 large button mushrooms, stems removed

    - 1/2 cup spinach, finely chopped

    - 1/4 cup feta cheese, crumbled

    - 1 tsp olive oil

    - Salt and pepper to taste

- Serves: 2

- Mode of cooking: Baking

- Procedure:

    1. Preheat oven to 375°F (190°C).

    2. In a bowl, mix spinach and feta cheese.

    3. Drizzle mushrooms with olive oil, salt, and pepper.

    4. Stuff each mushroom cap with the spinach and feta mixture.

    5. Place on a baking sheet and bake for 15-20 minutes or until mushrooms are tender.

- Nutritional Values: Approx. 100 calories, 5g protein, 7g fat, 4g carbohydrates.

Recipe 19: Zucchini Pizza Bites

- P.T.: 15 minutes

- Ingr.:

  - 1 zucchini, sliced into thick rounds

  - 1/4 cup marinara sauce (low sodium)

  - 1/4 cup shredded mozzarella cheese

  - Mini pepperoni slices or other toppings of choice

- Serves: 4

- Mode of cooking: Baking

- Procedure:

  1. Preheat oven to 400°F (200°C).

  2. Lay zucchini slices on a baking sheet.

  3. Spread a thin layer of marinara sauce on each slice.

  4. Sprinkle with mozzarella cheese and add toppings.

  5. Bake for 5-7 minutes or until cheese is melted and slightly golden.

- Nutritional Values: Approx. 80 calories, 5g protein, 4g fat, 6g carbohydrates.

Recipe 20: Coconut Almond Energy Balls

- P.T.: 20 minutes (+ chill time)

- Ingr.:

  - 1/2 cup almonds, finely chopped

  - 1/2 cup shredded coconut (unsweetened)

  - 2 tbsp honey or maple syrup

  - 1 tsp vanilla extract

- Serves: 10 (1 ball per serving)

- Mode of cooking: No-cook

- Procedure:

  1. In a mixing bowl, combine all ingredients until a sticky mixture forms.

  2. Using your hands, roll the mixture into small balls.

  3. Place on a parchment-lined tray and refrigerate for at least an hour before serving.

- Nutritional Values: Approx. 70 calories, 2g protein, 5g fat, 5g carbohydrates.

Satisfying dinners

Recipe 1: Lemon Herb Grilled Chicken

- P.T.: 25 minutes

- Ingr.:

  - 2 boneless, skinless chicken breasts

  - 1 lemon, zested and juiced

  - 2 tsp olive oil

  - 1 tsp fresh thyme, chopped

  - 1 tsp fresh rosemary, chopped

  - Salt and pepper to taste

- Serves: 2

- Mode of cooking: Grill

- Procedure:

  1. In a bowl, combine lemon zest, lemon juice, olive oil, thyme, rosemary, salt, and pepper.

  2. Marinate chicken breasts in the mixture for at least 15 minutes.

  3. Preheat grill to medium-high heat. Grill chicken for 6-7 minutes on each side or until cooked through.

  4. Serve with steamed vegetables.

- Nutritional values: Approx. 220 calories, 28g protein, 10g fat, 3g carbohydrates.

Recipe 2: Zucchini Noodle Stir-Fry

- P.T.: 20 minutes

- Ingr.:

  - 2 medium zucchinis, spiralized

  - 1/2 cup bell peppers, thinly sliced

  - 1/2 cup snap peas

  - 1/2 cup mushrooms, sliced

  - 2 tbsp soy sauce (low-sodium)

  - 1 tsp ginger, minced

- 1 garlic clove, minced

- 1 tbsp olive oil

- Serves: 2

- Mode of cooking: Sauté

- Procedure:

1. Heat oil in a pan over medium heat. Add garlic and ginger and sauté for 1 minute.

2. Add bell peppers, snap peas, and mushrooms. Cook for 4-5 minutes.

3. Add zucchini noodles and soy sauce, stir-frying for an additional 3-4 minutes.

4. Serve immediately.

- Nutritional values: Approx. 125 calories, 5g protein, 7g fat, 13g carbohydrates.

Recipe 3: Baked Salmon with Asparagus

- P.T.: 30 minutes

- Ingr.:

- 2 salmon fillets (4 oz each)

- 1 bunch asparagus, trimmed

- 1 tbsp olive oil

- 1 lemon, thinly sliced

- Salt and pepper to taste

- Serves: 2

- Mode of cooking: Bake

- Procedure:

1. Preheat oven to 375°F (190°C).

2. Arrange salmon fillets and asparagus on a baking sheet. Drizzle with olive oil.

3. Season with salt and pepper, and top salmon with lemon slices.

4. Bake for 20-25 minutes or until salmon is cooked through.

5. Serve immediately.

- Nutritional values: Approx. 270 calories, 25g protein, 15g fat, 5g carbohydrates.

Recipe 4: Spiced Turkey Lettuce Wraps

- P.T.: 20 minutes
- Ingr.:
  - 1/2 lb ground turkey
  - 1/2 cup red bell pepper, diced
  - 1/2 cup carrots, shredded
  - 2 green onions, chopped
  - 1 tbsp low-sodium soy sauce
  - 1 tsp ground cumin
  - 1 tsp paprika
  - 1 tsp chili powder
  - 4 large lettuce leaves
  - 1 tbsp olive oil
- Serves: 2
- Mode of cooking: Sauté
- Procedure:

1. Heat olive oil in a pan over medium heat. Add ground turkey, breaking it apart as it cooks.

2. Once turkey is almost cooked through, add bell pepper, carrots, and spices. Continue cooking until vegetables are tender.

3. Remove from heat and stir in green onions and soy sauce.

4. Spoon turkey mixture into lettuce leaves and serve.

- Nutritional values: Approx. 250 calories, 28g protein, 12g fat, 8g carbohydrates.

Recipe 5: Broccoli and Cauliflower Soup

- P.T.: 30 minutes
- Ingr.:
  - 1 cup broccoli, chopped
  - 1 cup cauliflower, chopped
  - 2 cups chicken broth (low-sodium)
  - 1/2 cup onions, diced

- 1 garlic clove, minced

  - 1 tsp olive oil

  - Salt and pepper to taste

- Serves: 2

 Mode of cooking: Simmer

- Procedure:

  1. In a pot, heat olive oil over medium heat. Add onions and garlic, sautéing until translucent.

  2. Add broccoli, cauliflower, and chicken broth. Bring to a boil.

  3. Reduce heat and simmer for 20 minutes or until vegetables are tender.

  4. Use a blender or immersion blender to puree the soup until smooth.

  5. Season with salt and pepper, then serve.

- Nutritional values: Approx. 90 calories, 4g protein, 3g fat, 12g carbohydrates.

Recipe 6: Grilled Tuna Steaks

- P.T.: 15 minutes

- Ingr.:

  - 2 tuna steaks (4 oz each)

  - 2 tsp olive oil

  - 1 tsp dried basil

  - 1 lemon, zested and juiced

  - Salt and pepper to taste

- Serves: 2

- Mode of cooking: Grill

- Procedure:

  1. In a bowl, mix olive oil, basil, lemon zest, lemon juice, salt, and pepper.

  2. Marinate tuna steaks for 10 minutes.

  3. Grill on high heat for 2-3 minutes on each side.

  4. Serve with steamed green beans.

- Nutritional values: Approx. 220 calories, 30g protein, 10g fat, 1g carbohydrates.

Recipe 7: Turkey and Veggie Stuffed Peppers

- P.T.: 40 minutes
- Ingr.:
  - 2 bell peppers, halved and seeds removed
  - 1/2 lb lean ground turkey
  - 1/2 cup zucchini, diced
  - 1/2 cup tomatoes, diced
  - 1/4 cup onions, diced
  - 1 garlic clove, minced
  - 1 tsp olive oil
- Salt and pepper to taste
- Serves: 2
- Mode of cooking: Bake
- Procedure:
  1. Preheat oven to 375°F (190°C).
  2. In a pan, heat olive oil over medium heat. Add onions and garlic, sautéing until translucent.
  3. Add ground turkey, breaking it apart. Cook until browned.
  4. Stir in zucchini and tomatoes. Season with salt and pepper.
  5. Fill bell pepper halves with turkey mixture. Place in a baking dish.
  6. Cover with foil and bake for 25-30 minutes or until peppers are tender.
  7. Serve hot.
- Nutritional values: Approx. 260 calories, 28g protein, 9g fat, 14g carbohydrates.

Recipe 8: Spinach and Feta Egg Muffins

- P.T.: 30 minutes
- Ingr.:
  - 4 large eggs
  - 1/2 cup fresh spinach, chopped
  - 1/4 cup feta cheese, crumbled
  - 1/4 cup red bell pepper, diced

- Salt and pepper to taste
- Serves: 4
- Mode of cooking: Bake
- Procedure:

  1. Preheat oven to 375°F (190°C).

  2. Whisk eggs in a bowl. Add spinach, feta, bell pepper, salt, and pepper. Mix well.

  3. Pour mixture into greased muffin tins.

  4. Bake for 20-25 minutes or until set.

  5. Serve warm.
- Nutritional values: Approx. 85 calories, 7g protein, 5g fat, 2g carbohydrates.

Recipe 9: Shrimp and Snow Pea Sauté

- P.T.: 15 minutes
- Ingr.:

  - 1/2 lb shrimp, peeled and deveined

  - 1 cup snow peas

  - 1 tbsp olive oil

  - 1 tsp ginger, minced

  - 1 garlic clove, minced

  - 2 tbsp low-sodium soy sauce
- Serves: 2
- Mode of cooking: Sauté
- Procedure:

  1. Heat olive oil in a pan over medium heat. Add ginger and garlic, sautéing for 1 minute.

  2. Add shrimp. Cook until they turn pink.

  3. Add snow peas and soy sauce. Sauté for another 2-3 minutes.

  4. Serve hot.
- Nutritional values: Approx. 180 calories, 24g protein, 7g fat, 5g carbohydrates.

Recipe 10: Cabbage and Chicken Salad

- P.T.: 15 minutes

- Ingr.:

  - 1 cup cooked chicken breast, shredded

  - 2 cups shredded cabbage

  - 1 carrot, julienned

  - 1/4 cup green onions, chopped

  - 2 tbsp apple cider vinegar

  - 1 tbsp olive oil

  - Salt and pepper to taste

- Serves: 2

- Mode of cooking: Mix

- Procedure:

  1. In a large bowl, combine chicken, cabbage, carrot, and green onions.

  2. In a separate small bowl, whisk together apple cider vinegar, olive oil, salt, and pepper.

  3. Pour dressing over the salad and toss to combine.

  4. Serve chilled.

- Nutritional values: Approx. 215 calories, 25g protein, 8g fat, 8g carbohydrates.

Recipe 11: Broiled Salmon with Asparagus

- P.T.: 20 minutes

- Ingr.:

  - 2 salmon fillets (4 oz each)

  - 10 asparagus spears, trimmed

  - 1 tbsp olive oil

  - 1 lemon, zested and juiced

  - Salt and pepper to taste

- Serves: 2

- Mode of cooking: Broil

- Procedure:

1. Preheat broiler.

2. In a bowl, mix olive oil, lemon zest, lemon juice, salt, and pepper.

3. Brush the mixture onto salmon fillets and asparagus.

4. Place salmon and asparagus on a baking sheet.

5. Broil for 7-8 minutes, or until salmon flakes easily.

6. Serve immediately.

- Nutritional values: Approx. 240 calories, 28g protein, 12g fat, 4g carbohydrates.

Recipe 12: Zucchini Noodle Stir-Fry with Chicken

- P.T.: 20 minutes

- Ingr.:

  - 1 cup cooked chicken breast, sliced

  - 2 medium zucchinis, spiralized into noodles

  - 1/2 red bell pepper, sliced

  - 1 tbsp olive oil

  - 2 tbsp low-sodium soy sauce

  - 1 garlic clove, minced

  - 1 tsp ginger, minced

- Serves: 2

- Mode of cooking: Sauté

- Procedure:

  1. Heat olive oil in a skillet over medium heat.

  2. Add garlic and ginger, sauté for 1 minute.

  3. Add chicken and bell pepper, cook for 3-4 minutes.

  4. Add zucchini noodles and soy sauce. Stir-fry for another 2-3 minutes.

  5. Serve hot.

- Nutritional values: Approx. 220 calories, 25g protein, 9g fat, 10g carbohydrates.

Recipe 13: Cauliflower Fried 'Rice'

- P.T.: 25 minutes
- Ingr.:
  - 2 cups cauliflower rice (grated cauliflower)
  - 1/2 cup peas and carrots mix, frozen
  - 2 eggs, beaten
  - 2 green onions, sliced
  - 2 tbsp low-sodium soy sauce
  - 1 tbsp olive oil
  - 1 tsp sesame oil
  - Serves: 2
- Mode of cooking: Sauté
- Procedure:

  1. Heat olive oil in a skillet over medium heat.

  2. Add peas and carrots mix, cook for 2-3 minutes.

  3. Push the vegetables to the side, pour eggs into the skillet. Scramble the eggs and combine with vegetables.

  4. Stir in cauliflower rice, green onions, and soy sauce. Cook for 5-7 minutes, stirring frequently.

  5. Drizzle with sesame oil.

  6. Serve hot.

- Nutritional values: Approx. 190 calories, 10g protein, 10g fat, 14g carbohydrates.

Recipe 14: Baked Cod with Spinach

- P.T.: 30 minutes
- Ingr.:
  - 2 cod fillets (4 oz each)
  - 2 cups fresh spinach
  - 1 tbsp olive oil
  - 1 garlic clove, minced
  - Salt and pepper to taste

- Lemon wedges for serving

- Serves: 2

- Mode of cooking: Bake

- Procedure:

1. Preheat oven to 375°F (190°C).

2. In a skillet, heat olive oil over medium heat. Add garlic and spinach, sauté until wilted.

3. Place a layer of sautéed spinach in a baking dish, then place cod fillets on top.

4. Season with salt and pepper.

5. Bake for 20-25 minutes or until cod flakes easily.

6. Serve with lemon wedges.

- Nutritional values: Approx. 210 calories, 28g protein, 8g fat, 2g carbohydrates.

Recipe 15: Beef Lettuce Wraps

- P.T.: 20 minutes

- Ingr.:

- 1/2 lb lean ground beef

- 1/4 cup red bell pepper, diced

- 1/4 cup carrots, julienned

- 8 lettuce leaves (e.g., iceberg or butter lettuce)

- 1 tbsp low-sodium soy sauce

- 1 tsp olive oil

- Serves: 2

- Mode of cooking: Sauté

- Procedure:

1. Heat olive oil in a skillet over medium heat.

2. Add ground beef, breaking it apart. Cook until browned.

3. Stir in bell pepper, carrots, and soy sauce. Cook for another 3-4 minutes.

4. Serve beef mixture in lettuce leaves, wrapping them like tacos.

- Nutritional values: Approx. 230 calories, 25g protein, 10g fat, 5g carbohydrates.

Recipe 16: Shrimp & Veggie Skewers

- P.T.: 25 minutes
- Ingr.:
  - 12 large shrimps, peeled and deveined
  - 1 red bell pepper, cut into squares
  - 1 zucchini, sliced
  - 1 tbsp olive oil
  - 1 lemon, zested and juiced
  - Salt and pepper to taste
  - Serves: 2
  - Mode of cooking: Grill or broil
- Procedure:
  1. Preheat grill or broiler.
  2. In a bowl, mix olive oil, lemon zest, lemon juice, salt, and pepper.
  3. Thread shrimps, bell pepper, and zucchini onto skewers.
  4. Brush the skewers with the oil and lemon mixture.
  5. Grill or broil for 6-8 minutes, turning occasionally until shrimps are pink.
  6. Serve immediately.
- Nutritional values: Approx. 180 calories, 20g protein, 8g fat, 6g carbohydrates.

Recipe 17: Spinach & Mushroom Omelette

- P.T.: 15 minutes
- Ingr.:
  - 3 large egg whites
  - 1/2 cup spinach, chopped
  - 1/4 cup mushrooms, sliced
  - 1 tbsp feta cheese, crumbled
  - 1 tsp olive oil
  - Salt and pepper to taste
- Serves: 1
- Mode of cooking: Sauté

- Procedure:

  1. Heat olive oil in a non-stick skillet over medium heat.

  2. Add mushrooms and sauté until soft.

  3. Add spinach and cook until wilted.

  4. In a bowl, whisk egg whites, salt, and pepper. Pour over vegetables in the skillet.

  5. After nearly setting, spread feta over one half of the omelette and fold it over the cheese.

  6. Provide hot.

- Nutritional values: Approx. 140 calories, 15g protein, 6g fat, 4g carbohydrates.

Recipe 18: Grilled Chicken Salad with Balsamic Vinaigrette

- P.T.: 25 minutes

- Ingr.:

  - 2 chicken breasts (4 oz each)

  - 4 cups mixed salad greens

  - 1/2 cucumber, sliced

  - 10 cherry tomatoes, halved

  - 1 tablespoons olive oil

  - 2 tbsp balsamic vinegar

  - Salt and pepper to taste

- Serves: 2

- Mode of cooking: Grill

- Procedure:

  1. Preheat grill.

  2. Season chicken with salt and pepper. Grill for 6-7 minutes each side, or until cooked through.

  3. In a bowl, whisk olive oil, balsamic vinegar, salt, and pepper.

  4. In a large bowl, toss salad greens, cucumber, and cherry tomatoes with the dressing.

5. Serve grilled chicken over the salad.

- Nutritional values: Approx. 260 calories, 30g protein, 10g fat, 8g carbohydrates.

Recipe 19: Tofu & Green Bean Stir-Fry

- P.T.: 20 minutes
- Ingr.:
  - 1 cup firm tofu, cubed
  - 1 cup green beans, trimmed
  - 2 tbsp low-sodium soy sauce
  - 1 garlic clove, minced
  - 1 tsp ginger, minced
  - 1 tsp olive oil
- Serves: 2
- Mode of cooking: Sauté
- Procedure:
  1. Heat olive oil in a skillet over medium heat.
  2. Add garlic and ginger, sauté for 1 minute.
  3. Add tofu cubes, cook until slightly golden.
  4. Add green beans and soy sauce, cook for another 4-5 minutes.
  5. Serve hot.
- Nutritional values: Approx. 150 calories, 12g protein, 7g fat, 8g carbohydrates.

Recipe 20: Turkey & Veggie Stuffed Peppers

- P.T.: 40 minutes
- Ingr.:
  - 2 bell peppers, halved and seeds removed
  - 1/2 lb lean ground turkey
  - 1/2 cup zucchini, diced
  - 1/4 cup onion, diced
  - 1/4 cup tomato sauce
  - 1 tsp olive oil

- Salt and pepper to taste

- Serves: 2

- Mode of cooking: Bake

- Procedure:

  1. Preheat oven to 375°F (190°C).

  2. In a skillet, heat olive oil over medium heat. Add onion and sauté until translucent.

  3. Add ground turkey, breaking it apart. Cook until browned.

  4. Stir in zucchini and tomato sauce. Cook for another 3-4 minutes.

  5. Stuff bell pepper halves with the turkey mixture.

  6. Place in a baking dish and cover with foil.

  7. Bake for 25-30 minutes or until peppers are tender.

  8. Serve hot.

- Nutritional values: Approx. 240 calories, 28g protein, 9g fat, 12g carbohydrates.

Chapter 6. Tips for Eating Out

Intro

For most of us residing in bustling metropolitan cities, social occasions are an integral part of life. They punctuate our daily routines, providing opportunities to bond, celebrate, and create cherished memories. But for those on a dedicated path to health and wellness, these events often come with a dose of apprehension. How does one navigate a spread of tempting foods while adhering to Dr. Nowzaradan's dietary principles? How do we strike a balance between enjoying the moment and making smart choices?

This chapter delves into the art of managing social occasions without compromising your dietary commitment. But remember, it's not about stringent restrictions or missing out on the fun. Instead, it's about making informed decisions that allow you to partake in the festivities wholeheartedly while staying true to your health goals. As we explore strategies for eating out, attending gatherings, or celebrating milestones, it becomes evident that with the right mindset and preparation, any social event can be both enjoyable and align with your wellness journey.

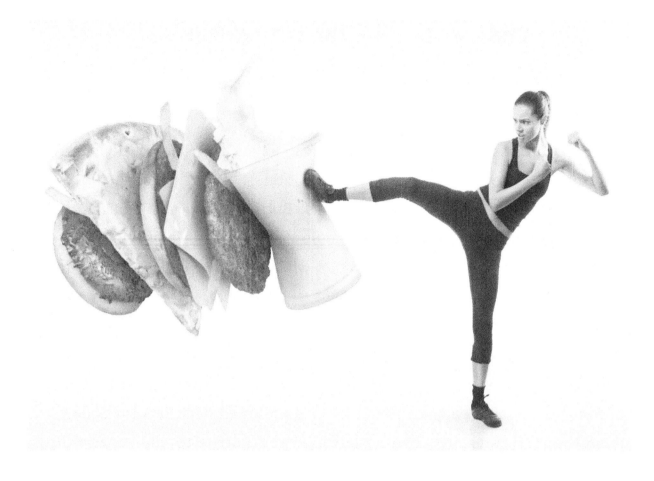

Smart choices at restaurants

Dining out is an integral part of our social lives. Whether celebrating a milestone, enjoying a date night, or simply taking a break from cooking, restaurants are where memories are made. But when one is trying to adhere to a diet, especially one as specific as Dr. Nowzaradan's, the plethora of choices can be daunting. So, how do you make smart decisions without compromising on the experience or the diet?

It's crucial to familiarize oneself with the menu before diving into the selections. At first glance, dishes might seem off-limits, but upon closer inspection, you might find viable options. For instance, while a creamy pasta dish might be an obvious dish to avoid, grilled fish or lean meats can be an excellent alternative. Seek out dishes where protein is at the forefront, as these will most likely align with the diet's high protein and low carbohydrate focus.

Never hesitate to engage with the server. They are there to ensure you have the best dining experience. If you're unsure about a particular dish's ingredients or how it's prepared, ask. By understanding what goes into each dish, you can make informed decisions.

Don't be shy about asking for modifications. Most restaurants are flexible and willing to accommodate specific dietary needs. For instance, if a dish comes with a heavy cream sauce, request it on the side or inquire if there's a lighter alternative. Similarly, if a meal comes with a carb-heavy side, such as fries or mashed potatoes, see if it's possible to substitute it with a salad or steamed vegetables.

Beverages can be a hidden source of excess calories. Opt for water, unsweetened iced tea, or sparkling water over sugary drinks or alcohol. If you do choose to indulge in an alcoholic beverage, opt for lighter choices like a glass of wine or a simple cocktail without sugary mixers.

Paying attention to the act of eating can make a world of difference. Savor each bite, chew thoroughly, and take your time. By eating slowly, you give your body the time it needs to recognize when it's full, which helps in preventing overeating.

We've all been there. The bread basket arrives, and before you know it, you've consumed more than intended. If you decide to indulge, limit yourself to a single piece and skip the butter or olive oil.

Appetizers can be a tricky territory. Many are fried or come with rich dips that can quickly add up in calories. If you're keen on starting with an appetizer, consider options like a fresh salad (with dressing on the side) or a broth-based soup. These choices can satiate initial hunger pangs without derailing your dietary goals.

Restaurant portions can be notably generous. Consider sharing a dish with a dining companion. This not only allows you to try different dishes but also ensures you don't overeat.

It's entirely possible to enjoy a sweet treat without going overboard. Opt for fruit-based desserts or those that don't come with heavy creams or syrups. Sharing a dessert is another excellent way to indulge without overcommitting.

Once your dining experience is over, take a moment to reflect on the choices you made. Celebrate the smart decisions, and if there were moments of indulgence, think about how you might approach them differently next time. Remember, every meal is a new opportunity to make choices that align with your goals.

In conclusion, dining out doesn't have to be a daunting experience for those following Dr. Nowzaradan's diet. With a bit of planning, asking the right questions, and making informed choices, you can enjoy a delightful meal without veering off the path to your health goals. So the next time you find yourself at a restaurant, remember these tips, and dine with confidence.

Managing social occasions

Life in urban metropolitan areas is woven with a rich tapestry of social events, from casual meetups to grand occasions. Whether it's a family wedding, a friend's birthday bash, or simply a weekend brunch, such gatherings pose unique challenges for anyone committed to a dietary path. Yet, maintaining Dr. Nowzaradan's philosophy during these events is not about isolation but integration. It's about finding the balance between enjoying these pivotal life moments and staying true to your wellness journey.

Every successful endeavor begins with the right mindset. Anticipate the event and remind yourself of its significance. Remember, these occasions are about connection, celebration, and shared experiences. It's essential to be present mentally, enjoying conversations and creating memories. The food, though a significant component, should not be the sole focus. Empower yourself with the thought that you are in control of your choices.

Familiarizing yourself with the event can work wonders. If it's at a venue you know, think about the typical food and drink served there. If not, a quick conversation with the host can provide insights. This simple step can help you anticipate possible menu options and make informed choices.

One of the most effective ways to ensure there's something you can enjoy without worry is to contribute to the meal. Bring a dish that aligns with your dietary requirements. It serves dual purposes: sharing a bit of your culinary skills with loved ones and ensuring there's something you can indulge in guilt-free.

Buffets are a common feature in many social occasions, and they present both a challenge and an opportunity. The variety on offer means there are likely options that fit within Dr. Nowzaradan's philosophy. Start by scanning the entire spread before taking anything. Prioritize protein-rich dishes and those abundant in fresh vegetables. Limit starchy sides and sauces which can often be calorie-dense. And always remember, just because it's all-you-can-eat doesn't mean you have to try everything.

There will invariably be well-meaning friends or relatives who'll insist you try "just a bite" of something that doesn't align with your dietary choices. Politely but firmly decline. A simple "I'm trying to eat a certain way for my health, but I appreciate the offer," often suffices.

In many cultures, drinking is synonymous with socializing. But alcohol can be a sneaky source of calories. If you choose to drink, opt for clear spirits with low-calorie mixers or a glass of wine. Consider setting a personal limit before the event begins. And always, intersperse alcoholic beverages with glasses of water.

If the occasion permits, dance! It's a fun way to burn off some of the extra calories you might consume. Not to mention, it's a great way to interact, enjoy the event, and get a mini workout.

Let's be real: there might be times you overindulge. Instead of berating yourself, accept it as a part of the journey. Every meal is an independent event. One indulgent meal doesn't define your entire dietary journey. Recognize it, learn from it, and move on.

After a night of socializing, give yourself a pat on the back for the smart choices you made. If there were lapses, consider them learning moments, not failures. The next day, return to your regular eating habits. You might even consider engaging in a bit more physical activity to balance out any extra intake.

Ultimately, social events are but a small fraction of our lives. They're moments of joy, laughter, and connection. By managing these occasions effectively, you not only take care of your health but also ensure that these memories are free of regret and guilt. Remember, the journey to a healthier you is not about perfection but persistence. Every social occasion successfully navigated brings you one step closer to your goal, allowing you to relish life's beautiful moments in the best of health.

Conclusion

Navigating the landscape of social occasions while maintaining dietary discipline is undoubtedly a challenge, yet not an insurmountable one. As this chapter has illuminated, the key lies in preparation, a proactive approach, and a clear understanding of one's priorities. By adopting the strategies and insights provided, you can confidently attend any event, savoring the experience without the shadow of dietary guilt.

In essence, managing social occasions on Dr. Nowzaradan's plan is a reflection of the broader journey towards health and well-being. It's about recognizing that each choice, while seemingly small in the moment, contributes to a larger mosaic of a healthier, happier you. The joy of social gatherings need not be at odds with your commitment to wellness. With the right tools and mindset, they can harmoniously coexist, allowing you to live fully, celebrate freely, and eat wisely. As you move forward, embrace these moments not as hurdles, but as opportunities to reinforce your dedication, resilience, and growth.

Chapter 7. Physical Exercise and Dr. Nowzaradan's Plan

Intro

The gleaming skyscrapers of the city, casting long shadows as the sun sets, bear witness to myriad stories. Among them is the collective journey of urbanites seeking more than just a thriving career or social life; they chase well-being, the melding of mind and body into an oasis of health. Amid the orchestrated chaos of city life, Dr. Nowzaradan's holistic approach offers a resounding note of clarity. It's not merely about the food we eat but also the lives we lead and the movement we incorporate.

Movement, in essence, is life. Each step we take, whether it's on the bustling streets, in the serene confines of a park, or within the sacred space of our homes, speaks of our innate need to be active. The human body, a marvel of nature, is designed to move, to flex, to dance, to run. However, in the urban sprawl where time becomes a luxury and schedules are packed, integrating regular physical activity often takes a back seat.

Before venturing further, a note of caution is paramount. As Dr. Nowzaradan's plan unfurls, it emphasizes the individuality of health. Each person's journey is unique, shaped by their experiences, biology, and circumstances. Consequently, before diving headfirst into any fitness regimen, it's crucial to ensure your health aligns with the demands of the routine. The cornerstone of any sustainable fitness journey is the knowledge of one's own body. Seek professional advice, undergo necessary medical checks, and ensure you're stepping onto this path with informed confidence.

Dr. Nowzaradan is an advocate of balance. His plan is not about extreme measures but sustainable changes that blend seamlessly into the fabric of daily life. One of the pillars of his approach is the recommendation of at least 30 minutes of physical activity each day. Think of it as an investment, not in the fleeting currency of physical aesthetics but in the enduring wealth of health and well-being.

The importance of physical activity in weight loss

On the bustling streets of metropolitan cities, where skyscrapers touch the heavens and life never takes a breather, it's easy to find oneself wrapped up in the hustle and neglecting the essential: our health. As we journey through the ever-evolving tapestry of life, the significance of intertwining physical activity with our daily routines becomes glaringly apparent, especially in our pursuit of weight loss.

For many, the idea of weight loss is heavily synonymous with diet, nutrition, and the foods we consume. This perception isn't entirely misplaced. However, the story is incomplete without the pivotal chapter on physical activity. Just as a painter needs both colors and canvas, or a musician requires notes and rhythm, weight loss demands both diet and exercise. They complement each other, crafting a symphony of wellness that resonates with vitality.

Our bodies, intricate and wondrous in design, are built for movement. Every step taken, every muscle flexed, fuels the burning of calories. But what does this mean in the context of weight loss? It's simple, really. Weight loss transpires when the body expends more calories than it consumes. While managing our calorie intake through diet plays a monumental role, increasing calorie expenditure via physical activity accelerates the process.

Let's take a closer look. When we engage in exercise, especially strength training, we not only burn calories during the actual activity but also elevate our resting metabolic rate. This phenomenon is called excess post-exercise oxygen consumption (EPOC), often termed the 'afterburn effect'. Simply put, after an intense workout session, our bodies continue to burn calories at an elevated rate even while resting.

Moreover, consistent exercise fosters muscle growth. Muscle tissue, by nature, is metabolically active. The more muscle mass one has, the more calories they burn at rest. This means that by cultivating muscle, we transform our bodies into more efficient calorie-burning machines.

But physical activity's role in weight loss isn't limited to mere mathematics of calorie counting. It's a holistic experience, touching every facet of our well-being. Exercise releases endorphins, those magical chemicals in our brain that act as natural painkillers and mood elevators. This not only makes us feel good post-workout but also bolsters our motivation, helping us maintain consistency in our weight loss journey.

Another profound impact of physical activity lies in its ability to combat stress. Urban living, with its relentless pace, often engenders stress, a silent adversary to weight loss. Stress triggers the release of the hormone cortisol, which in turn can promote fat storage, especially around the abdominal region. Regular physical activity mitigates stress, curbing cortisol levels and its counterproductive effects on weight loss.

In the grand theater of weight loss, diet sets the stage, but exercise delivers the performance. They are co-stars in this production, and sidelining one does injustice to the other. Consider this analogy: if dieting alone is like trying to light a damp matchstick, then combining it with exercise ensures the flame not only catches but blazes brilliantly.

For those in metropolitan cities, with gyms at every corner and parks sprawling with jogging paths, integrating physical activity can be both convenient and enjoyable. Whether it's a morning run as the city awakens, a yoga class during lunch break, or a dance session under the neon-lit skyline, the opportunities are abundant and diverse.

However, it's essential to remember that while exercise aids weight loss, it's not a free pass to indulge without restraint. It's a partnership where both diet and exercise share equal responsibility. Overcompensating with excessive food intake after a workout can negate the calorie deficit created, stalling weight loss progress. Physical activity, in its myriad forms, is a beacon of hope, illuminating the path to weight loss. It challenges us, reshapes us, and infuses us with an energy that's both invigorating and transformative. In the words of the renowned Dr. Nowzaradan, "It's not about perfect, it's about effort." So, every time you lace up those sneakers, remember, you're not just burning calories; you're kindling the flame of a healthier, more vibrant you.

Tips for starting and maintaining a routine

Downtown, the hum of a thriving metropolis teems with the symphony of honking cars, fervent chatter, and the distant beat of a subway train. Amid the city's unstoppable rhythm, there's a pulse—a collective heartbeat that thrives on movement and progress. For urbanites seeking to rekindle their personal vigor, starting an exercise routine can be transformative. But in a world of endless tasks and time ticking away, how does one integrate a consistent fitness regime?

The heart of any journey begins with understanding one's reasons. Why do you want to start an exercise routine? Is it to shed those extra pounds? Or perhaps to relish the vitality of being able to dance at a party without losing breath? By recognizing the 'why', we set a foundation that can weather moments of doubt.

For many, embarking on this journey is about reclaiming oneself, reshaping not just the physique but the narrative of personal well-being. Starting isn't a declaration of war against one's body but rather an act of love, a commitment to oneself.

Every individual's rhythm is as unique as their fingerprint. Some may resonate with the calm of yoga during sunrise, while others find solace in the adrenaline-pumping beats of a late-night spin class. It's crucial to explore various physical activities to discern what clicks. Perhaps it's the dance class that makes you feel alive, or the strength training session that leaves you feeling empowered. Whatever it may be, when you find that connection, you're more likely to stick to it.

In the luminous glow of motivation, it's tempting to pledge an hour at the gym every day or to run five miles at dawn. But when reality dawns, such lofty goals can become overwhelming, leading to early burnout. Instead, initiate with modest, attainable goals. If you're new to exercise, perhaps start with a fifteen-minute brisk walk thrice a week and gradually escalate from there. Celebrate the small victories; they compound into significant achievements.

In the maze of urban life, days blend into nights, and before we know it, weeks have passed. To prevent exercise from becoming a fleeting thought, rope in a workout buddy. Whether it's a friend, a colleague, or even a family member, having someone to share the journey can provide that extra push on days when motivation wanes. Additionally, sharing progress, challenges, and milestones can add a layer of joy and determination.

While establishing a routine is pivotal, it's equally vital to recognize that life is unpredictable. Some days the rain may pour, making that evening jog impossible. On others, work might extend into late hours, leaving no time for the gym. Rather than seeing these as setbacks, embrace them as opportunities to be adaptable. Maybe you can't go for a jog, but you could do a short indoor workout. Or perhaps you can incorporate activity into your day, like taking the stairs instead of the elevator.

A common misconception is that one needs to exercise with high intensity to see results. While challenging workouts have their place, it's the consistency over time that carves the path to transformation. Instead of focusing on the intensity of each workout, concentrate on maintaining regularity. A moderate but consistent routine can often yield more sustainable results than sporadic bursts of extreme activity.

The beauty of living in an urban sprawl is the myriad opportunities to incorporate movement. Instead of hailing a cab for a short distance, consider walking. Those moments when you're waiting for your coffee? Do some calf raises. Watching your favorite show? Incorporate some stretches. Every bit adds up, making fitness not an isolated task but an integrated lifestyle.

There will be days when the allure of the couch seems unbeatable. For such moments, having a source of inspiration can be the nudge you need. Maybe it's a motivational quote on your mirror or a playlist that invigorates your spirit. Remembering the testimonials of others, who've walked this path, can also serve as a powerful reminder of what's achievable.

Often, in the rush to reach the finish line, we forget to honor the journey. Every time you push your boundaries, whether it's an extra rep, an added minute, or even just showing up on a tough day, it's a victory. Celebrate these moments. They are the mosaic pieces in your transformative journey, each one adding color and shape to your evolving story.

The streets of the city, alive with their energy, reflect a truth about human nature—movement is life. In the narrative of weight loss and wellness, physical activity is not merely a chapter but a recurring theme. Starting and maintaining a routine, especially amidst urban chaos, can seem daunting. But with intention, adaptability, and consistent effort, every stride, jump, or dance becomes a step towards a healthier, more radiant self.

Conclusion

As our journey through the intricacies of Dr. Nowzaradan's plan comes to a close in this chapter, a few key takeaways resonate. The metropolitan cities, with their ebb and flow, represent the dynamic nature of life. To thrive amidst this dynamism, one must adapt, evolve, and, most importantly, move. Physical activity, as underscored in this chapter, isn't merely a route to weight loss. It's a bridge to holistic wellness, a tonic for the mind, body, and spirit.

The commitment to move every day, even if it's for just 30 minutes, is akin to a silent promise, a pact with oneself. It's a nod to the future, assuring better health, enhanced mood, and a zest for life. Dr. Nowzaradan's prescription of daily movement isn't a rigid dictum but a flexible guideline. It can manifest as a brisk walk, a dance session, yoga, or any activity that resonates with one's soul.

However, as one embarks on this invigorating path, a consistent reminder is essential: listen to your body. Each person's threshold and capacity differ. While pushing boundaries can lead to growth, it's equally important to recognize when to rest. And, as always, prior to embarking on any exercise regimen, ensure that your health permits it. Physical activity should be an avenue of joy, not a source of undue strain.

Dr. Nowzaradan's emphasis on the harmony of diet and exercise carves a roadmap for sustained well-being. As urban dwellers, the challenges are plenty, but so are the opportunities. Every staircase, park, and even living room becomes a potential arena for movement. Embrace it, celebrate it, and let each step be a testament to your commitment to health.

Chapter 8. Tackling Common Obstacles and Challenges

Intro

Stepping into the labyrinth of self-improvement is an act of bravery. Just as an adventurer is bound to face hurdles on his quest for treasure, so too will you come across challenges in your journey towards a healthier version of yourself. The vibrant pulse of metropolitan life, with its dazzling array of delicacies and distractions, serves as both a test and testament to our resolve. This chapter doesn't just acknowledge these tests, but embraces them, delving deep into the very nature of temptations and setbacks that are as inherent to urban life as the skyline itself. Before venturing into strategies and soulful contemplations, it's essential to equip ourselves with a broader perspective: understanding why these obstacles exist and recognizing their transformative power.

Navigating through the city's twists and turns, we're bound to face the sirens of temptation whether it's the beckoning aroma of a bakery, the allure of a cozy cafe, or the simple comfort of old habits. Yet, just as a city's charm lies not in its skyscrapers but the stories they hold, our journey's value isn't in the destination but the growth along the way. Setbacks, those little detours, can teach us more about ourselves than a straightforward journey ever could. They show us our vulnerabilities, test our determination, and, most importantly, give us a chance to rise stronger, wiser, and more resolute.

In the sections that follow, we'll unravel the emotional tapestry behind temptations, understand the psychology of setbacks, and arm ourselves with strategies to navigate them. While the urban jungle poses its challenges, it also offers the resilience of its spirit, a spirit that each one of us can harness.

Overcoming weight loss plateaus

In the heart of every metropolitan city, change is the only constant. Buildings grow taller, roads stretch further, and every corner evolves with time. As dwellers of these ever-evolving urban environments, we too are in a state of continuous transformation, especially when we commit to a healthier lifestyle. Every effort put into mindful eating and diligent exercise draws us closer to our ideal self. But, much like the occasional traffic jam in our bustling cities, there are moments in our journey towards optimal health where progress seems to halt: the dreaded weight loss plateau.

The weight loss plateau, while a common adversary for many on a wellness journey, can be likened to a red traffic light. It's not a sign to make a U-turn or park indefinitely; rather, it's a brief pause, a moment to recalibrate and reevaluate before moving forward once again.

At the beginning of a weight loss journey, enthusiasm runs high, and initial results are often rapid. This is primarily because, in the initial stages, the body sheds water weight. But as time progresses, the rate of weight loss tends to slow down, even if you're sticking to your dietary and exercise plan. This phenomenon is not a result of doing anything wrong; it's a natural adaptation by the body.

As we lose weight, our metabolism — the engine that burns calories to keep our body running— can decrease. With fewer pounds to carry around, the body simply doesn't need as much energy as it did before. So, with a reduced caloric need and a consistent caloric intake, weight loss naturally stalls.

It's early morning, the city is awakening, and as you stand at your window overlooking the urban sprawl, a feeling of stagnation washes over you. Those consistent numbers on the scale, despite all your efforts, can be disheartening. Here, the challenge is as much mental as it is physical.

It's easy to be lured into negative self-talk. Thoughts like "Maybe this is just how I'm meant to be" or "I've tried everything, and nothing's working" might start to dominate. But remember, every skyscraper that dots the city's skyline faced challenges during its construction. Yet, they stand tall, not because the process was easy, but because the vision was clear and the foundation strong.

In a world obsessed with numbers, it's natural to measure progress by the digits on the scale. But true wellness encompasses more than weight alone. Instead of solely focusing on weight, shift the focus to how you feel. Are you more energetic? Do your clothes fit better? Are you sleeping more soundly or finding everyday tasks easier to perform? These non-scale victories are essential indicators of progress and are often overlooked.

Strategies to Break Through

Much like finding alternate routes in a traffic jam, there are various strategies to overcome a weight loss plateau:

1. *Reassess Caloric Needs*: As you lose weight, your caloric needs change. It might be beneficial to consult a nutritionist or use online tools to gauge your new requirements.

2. *Change Up Your Routine*: Just as monotony can bore the mind, the body too craves variety. If you've been doing the same workout, consider mixing things up. Try a new exercise class or add intervals to your jogging routine.

3. *Strength Training*: Building muscle can give your metabolism a boost as muscle burns more calories at rest than fat. Consider incorporating strength training exercises into your regimen.

4. **Stay Hydrated**: Water plays a pivotal role in metabolism. Ensure you're drinking enough throughout the day.

5. **Rest and Recover**: Overexertion can lead to fatigue and even injury. Ensure you're giving your body ample time to recover between workouts.

If you've tried multiple strategies and still find yourself stagnant, it may be time to seek professional advice. A nutritionist or personal trainer can provide personalized guidance tailored to your needs. Additionally, underlying medical conditions could be at play, so consulting a physician might be necessary.

Every urbanite knows that the city's pulse is undeterred by challenges. Likewise, in the journey of wellness, plateaus are mere pauses, not endpoints. With understanding, strategy, and persistence, you can navigate this phase and emerge stronger, ready to continue your journey towards your healthiest self.

The weight loss plateau is not a reflection of failure, but rather an invitation. An invitation to dig deeper, to learn more about your body, and to refine your approach. In the grand tapestry of your wellness journey, it's but a single thread, woven intricately among countless successes. Remember, every challenge faced and overcome only adds to the richness of your story. So, take a deep breath, recalibrate, and drive forward with renewed determination.

Handling temptations and setbacks

In the shimmering heartbeats of the modern metropolitan, there's an undeniable allure that draws us in. The neon lights beckon, and the city pulses with promises. Life here is a sumptuous banquet of opportunities and experiences, and in the midst of it all, each of us attempts to find our own rhythm, our own balance. Just as the city presents diversions at every turn, so too does our journey to a healthier self. The roads to wellness are lined with temptations and dotted with setbacks. And navigating these challenges requires an understanding heart, a mindful approach, and an unwavering spirit.

To understand temptation is to recognize that it is deeply human. It isn't simply about craving a decadent dessert or yearning to skip a workout after a long day. Temptation is as much about our emotional and psychological state as it is about the object of our desire.

The City's Sirens: Think of that upscale bakery that just opened around the corner or the aroma wafting from a food truck during lunch hours. The city offers a buffet of delectable delights, each more tantalizing than the last. But more than the taste, these temptations often carry the weight of memories, the warmth of nostalgia, or the allure of novelty.

Emotional Currents: Often, we're drawn to indulgences not just for their sensory appeal but for the emotional comfort they promise. That chocolate cake isn't just dessert; it's a salve on a rough day, a celebration, a memory.

Setbacks. Those days when, despite our best intentions, we yield to temptation. Maybe it's a weekend of overindulgence or a week when life's chaos leaves no room for workouts. It's essential to understand that setbacks aren't failures; they're merely stumbles on a journey that's inherently challenging.

Acceptance Before Action: Before we can move past a setback, we must first accept it. Denial or excessive guilt doesn't propel us forward. Acceptance acknowledges our humanity, our imperfections, and it's the first step toward course correction.

The Resilience of the Urban Spirit: Much like the city that rebuilds after every storm, our spirit too has an innate resilience. Every setback is an opportunity to harness this strength, to rise, rebuild, and resume our journey.

Crafting a Temptation Strategy

Recognizing temptation is half the battle; the other half lies in crafting strategies to navigate it.

Delay, Don't Deny: When temptation beckons, instead of an outright denial, delay your response. Tell yourself, "I'll wait for 10 minutes." Often, this simple pause diminishes the intensity of the craving.

Understand Your Triggers: Are you more likely to snack when stressed? Do weekends derail your diet? Recognizing your unique triggers allows you to devise targeted strategies.

Positive Substitution: If you're craving something sweet, could fresh fruit or a small piece of dark chocolate satisfy that craving? Substituting a temptation with a healthier alternative often strikes the right balance.

Visualize the Aftermath: Before giving in to temptation, take a moment to visualize how you'll feel afterward. The immediate pleasure often pales in comparison to the lingering feelings of regret.

A single setback doesn't define your journey, but how you handle it can shape your path.

Practice Self-compassion: Speak to yourself as you would to a dear friend. Understand that everyone has off days. What's crucial is to not let one off day become an off week or month.

Revisit Your Why: Remember the reasons you started this journey. Whether it's fitting into a beloved dress, improving health markers, or simply feeling more vibrant, reconnecting with your 'why' can reignite your motivation.

Seek Support: Sharing your feelings with someone you trust can be therapeutic. Whether it's friends, family, or a support group, remember you're not alone.

In local theater, amidst the allure of neon lights and the symphony of bustling streets, our journey towards wellness is a deeply personal narrative. It's a tale of dreams, challenges, stumbles, and triumphs. And as with any great story, it's the challenges that add depth, the stumbles that make the rise more triumphant.
Temptations and setbacks aren't roadblocks; they're waypoints. They don't signify the end but offer moments of reflection, recalibration, and growth. In your quest for a healthier, happier self, may you navigate these challenges with grace, understanding, and an indomitable spirit that mirrors the resilient heart of the city you call home.

Conclusion

As the sun sets over our metropolitan sanctuary, casting its golden hues over skyscrapers and streets alike, we're reminded of the cyclical nature of life. Days turn into nights, seasons change, and we, amidst it all, evolve. This chapter, in its essence, is a celebration of that evolution. It's an ode to our stumbles, our vulnerabilities, and our triumphant returns. The city, with its myriad temptations and challenges, is not an adversary but a mentor, teaching us the value of resilience, patience, and self-awareness.

Temptations, as we've discovered, aren't just about the allure of the forbidden but a reflection of our emotional states, our memories, and our desires. By understanding them, we're not just avoiding a misstep but gaining insights into our psyche. Similarly, setbacks, those unwelcome pauses, are opportunities in disguise. They offer us a mirror, reflecting both our strengths and areas of growth.

As you continue your journey, remember that every city, no matter how sprawling, has its tranquil spots. Places where one can pause, reflect, and rejuvenate. In your quest for a healthier self, find those spaces within your soul. Celebrate your victories, learn from your detours, and most importantly, cherish the journey.

In the vast tapestry of life, it's not the destination but the stories, the experiences, and the growth that add color, depth, and beauty. Here's to your story, your journey, and the countless adventures that await in the heart of the city and within your soul.

Chapter 9. Success Stories: Testimonials from Those Who Followed the Plan

Intro

Amid the luminous skyline and ceaseless heartbeat of the urban metropolis, life often unfolds like a beautifully complex mosaic. Every individual becomes a piece of this intricate puzzle, driven by ambitions, aspirations, and challenges. The city's rhythm, marked by its fast pace and multitude of temptations, is exciting but can also pose unique challenges to one's health and well-being. But among these challenges emerge tales of hope, resilience, and transformation that inspire countless others to take a leap of faith towards a healthier tomorrow.

In the vast urban sprawl, it's easy to be swept away by the conveniences and indulgences the city offers. The delectable aroma wafting from a local bakery, the seductive allure of gourmet cuisines, the glamorous social gatherings around every corner – all these become integral elements of the city dweller's life. While these experiences add richness and depth to our lives, they also bring with them potential pitfalls for those aiming to maintain a healthy lifestyle. Temptations are abundant, and before one even realizes it, the balance between indulgence and well-being can tip.

However, every coin has two sides. While the urban jungle offers temptations, it also presents inspiring tales of individuals who, against all odds, transformed their lives by embracing health, wellness, and positivity. These are not just stories of weight loss; these are tales of individuals reclaiming their identities, of rediscovering their love for themselves and the world around them. Their journeys, marked by determination, struggles, and eventual success, provide a beacon of hope for many navigating the challenges of city life.

This chapter aims to shed light on such uplifting stories. It's not about statistics, dietary specifics, or exercise routines. It's about real people, just like you, who embarked on a journey with Dr. Nowzaradan's plan amidst the challenges of urban living. It's about Julia, who faced the daily temptations of a bakery right across her workplace; it's about Mark, whose love for gourmet cuisine led him down a path of imbalance, and Layla, whose passion for music became both her challenge and her redemption.

These tales are bound by a common thread - the journey towards a healthier self, aided by a comprehensive plan that takes into account not just dietary needs, but the myriad challenges posed by the urban environment. As you delve deeper into their accounts, you'll find reflections of your own experiences, struggles, and aspirations. Their stories become mirrors, allowing you to see your potential, recognize the hurdles, and believe in the possibility of transformation.

With each narrative, a pattern emerges, a testament to the adaptability of the human spirit. Whether it's the aroma of pastries that Julia learned to resist, Mark's culinary adventures that took a healthier turn, or Layla's rediscovery of her rhythm, these stories showcase that with the right guidance, unwavering determination, and a touch of self-love, one can turn the tide, even in the ever-demanding urban setting.

As you immerse yourself in these tales, remember that they're not outliers or exceptions. They are proof of the attainable, of what's possible when one decides to take charge. They remind us that transformation isn't just about the destination, but the journey – a journey marked by small choices, daily challenges, moments of doubt, and triumphant milestones.

Welcome to a chapter filled with inspiration, resilience, and most importantly, hope. Welcome to the tales of urban warriors who, with the aid of Dr. Nowzaradan's plan, scripted their success stories. Let their journeys illuminate your path, as you embark on your own voyage towards a healthier, happier self.

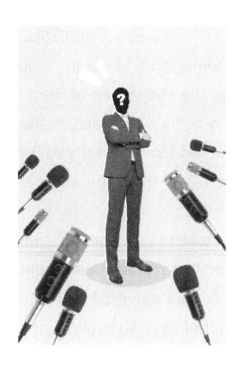

Interviews and accounts from those who succeeded with the diet

In the bustling heart of urban life, where time moves as swiftly as the passing trains and diets come and go like fleeting fashion trends, there exist tales of transformation that resonate with hope and determination. These stories aren't just about weight loss; they're about reclaiming life, about triumphs in the face of trials, and about the indomitable human spirit that arises from the challenges of metropolitan living.

Rebirth in the City: Julia's Journey

Julia, a 45-year-old magazine editor from New York City, recalls her first steps on this transformative path. The city, she said, had always felt like a double-edged sword. While it offered her opportunities and a dynamic career, it also presented countless temptations that impacted her health.

"I'd step out of my office, and there'd be this lovely bakery right across," Julia recalls, her voice tinged with nostalgia. "The sugary aroma, the inviting pastries, it was so easy to get drawn in. But over the years, it became more than just an occasional treat; it became a daily habit."

It wasn't just the pastries. Late-night work events, weekend brunches, and the ceaseless rhythm of city life pushed her into a cycle of unhealthy choices. Yet, it was during one such event, amidst the clinking glasses and soft murmur of conversations, that she overheard someone talk about Dr. Nowzaradan's plan.

"I remember feeling desperate, wanting to break free from the weight that had become both physical and emotional," she says. Embracing the diet, Julia found herself not only navigating through her nutritional choices but also rediscovering her relationship with food. Over the months, as the city bloomed and wilted with the changing seasons, so did Julia bloom into her best self, shedding not just pounds but also her apprehensions.

Rediscovering Love: Mark's Awakening

Mark, a 53-year-old architect, always had a penchant for gourmet cuisine. Living in San Francisco, he would often traverse the hills and valleys of the city, exploring its culinary delights. Yet, in this quest, he lost sight of balance. By the time he turned 50, Mark found himself burdened, both physically and mentally.

"There was a day," Mark pauses, gathering his thoughts, "when I realized I was breathless, just playing with my daughter in the park. It was a wake-up call."

When he started with Dr. Nowzaradan's plan, he initially struggled. "The city, with its myriad flavors, felt like an unending maze of temptations," he says. But with perseverance, Mark started finding joy in healthier alternatives. Gradually, he wasn't just eating to satiate his gourmet inclinations but to nourish his body and soul. Today, Mark not only relishes his meals but also every moment with his daughter, feeling fitter and more present than ever.

Dancing to a New Beat: Layla's Revival

Chicago's vibrant music scene was where Layla, a 38-year-old music instructor, found her passion and purpose. However, amid the rhythms and beats of the city's pulsating heart, she lost her own rhythm to a sedentary lifestyle and unhealthy eating habits.

"I felt trapped in a loop," Layla shares. "Being overweight affected my confidence, my teaching, and even my relationship with music."

Upon a friend's recommendation, she embarked on Dr. Nowzaradan's diet. "It was like learning a new musical piece, challenging yet exhilarating," she muses. As days turned to weeks and weeks to months, Layla not only shed weight but found a renewed passion for her art. Today, she dances and sways to her city's beats, a living testament to the transformative power of commitment.

Concluding Thoughts

Julia, Mark, and Layla are but a few stories amidst a sea of success tales, each echoing the challenges of urban living yet shining with hope, determination, and an undying spirit. Their experiences remind us that no matter the trials or temptations of city life, with the right guidance and a dash of perseverance, we can script our own tales of triumph. As they reclaimed their lives, so can you. Their stories aren't just tales; they're beacons, illuminating the path for all those seeking a healthier, more fulfilling life in the heart of the metropolis.

Chapter 10. Final Tips and Maintaining the Ideal Weight

Intro

The vibrant hum of a metropolitan city resonates with countless tales of ambition, dreams, challenges, and evolution. Just as the city is in a perpetual state of metamorphosis, so are its denizens, constantly seeking betterment, balance, and, in many cases, a return to holistic well-being. Our journey within these pages has mirrored the city's trajectory – dynamic, transformative, and intensely rewarding. As we delve into the final chapter of this enlightening expedition, we don't merely focus on the culmination of efforts, but on the synthesis of all that we've imbibed and how it paves the road ahead.

In the midst of urban chaos, finding tranquility and equilibrium, especially concerning health, becomes paramount. The gleaming facades of skyscrapers, the blaring horns of the bustling streets, the myriad colors of urban life - all these form the backdrop to a modern quest: the pursuit of health and the maintenance of one's ideal weight. The path you've trodden so far is reflective of the city's labyrinthine alleys – sometimes straightforward, occasionally confounding, but always leading to revelations.

If the preceding chapters were the intricate blueprints, laying the foundation and erecting the pillars of a healthier life, consider this chapter as the rooftop garden – a place of reflection, consolidation, and forward vision. We've addressed the science, unraveled the strategies, and equipped you with tools. Now, it's time to gaze upon the skyline of your achievements and plot the horizons you're yet to conquer.

Weight, much like the ever-ticking clock in a town square, is but a metric, a reference point. The real narrative lies in the pages between the starting line and this moment. It's in the transformation tales whispered in the hushed tones of midnight conversations, the silent battles won over temptations, and the joyous rhythm of newfound energy. As we embark on this chapter, it's time to reflect, not just on the scales and numbers but on the person you've become and the bright, boundless path that lies ahead.

How to maintain long-term weight

For many living amidst the hustle and bustle of a metropolitan city, the journey to weight loss and achieving that ideal number on the scale can feel like a triumphant final scene in a hard-fought movie. The applause is loud, the scene is radiant, and the protagonist, after countless obstacles, finally stands victorious. But what the movies often don't show is the sequel – the journey after the goal is reached, where maintaining that victory becomes the next challenge.

In the vibrant urban setting, with its myriad temptations and fast-paced lifestyle, maintaining weight is more of an art than a mere follow-up act. It requires as much dedication, if not more, as the initial weight loss journey. So how does one master this art amidst the skyscrapers, gourmet restaurants, and ever-evolving culinary temptations? Let's delve into the secrets of long-term weight maintenance.

Your body, after undergoing a significant transformation, has found a new equilibrium. Recognizing this "new normal" is vital. You are no longer in the active phase of shedding pounds but transitioning into a phase where you'll have to adopt a balanced approach to keep those pounds off.

In a city renowned for its diverse culinary palette, every street and corner can feel like a gastronomic adventure waiting to unfold. But being mindful of what you eat becomes crucial. Every bite matters. It's not about denying yourself the pleasures of urban cuisine but rather about making conscious choices. Opt for that grilled salmon over the creamy pasta or choose the fresh fruit tart over the triple-layered chocolate cake.

Consistency is the Key

The metropolitan life is unpredictable. Late-night work shifts, impromptu social gatherings, or weekend getaways can sometimes throw a wrench in your routine. However, the key is to remain consistent. If you miss a day of exercise, make it up the next day. If you indulged a bit at a party, ensure the next few meals are balanced and nutritious.

The urban landscape, with its skyscrapers and bustling streets, can be your playground. Opt for walking to your nearby cafe instead of taking a cab. Use the stairs in your office building. Participate in community yoga sessions in the park. The city offers countless opportunities for you to stay active, embrace them.

It's easy to lose track amidst the urban chaos. Having regular check-ins, be it through a journal, an app, or with your nutritionist, can help keep you on track. It's not about obsessing over every ounce but ensuring you're on the right path.

Living in a metropolis often means life is grand and fast. But when it comes to weight maintenance, it's the small victories that count. Did you choose a salad over fries? Did you opt for a brisk walk instead of binge-watching a show? Every small choice contributes to the bigger picture.

The urban world is ever-evolving, with new dietary trends, fitness regimes, and health tips emerging every day. Stay informed. If a new health trend aligns with your goals and feels right, don't hesitate to incorporate it into your routine.

The metropolitan city, with its millions, offers you a chance to connect with those on the same journey. Join support groups, attend workshops, or simply find a fitness buddy. Sharing experiences, challenges, and tips can provide the motivation you need.

Your body is your best guide. It will give you signals when things are amiss. If you feel unusually fatigued, hungrier than normal, or just out of sync, it's a cue to re-evaluate and adjust.

Remember, reaching your ideal weight isn't the end; it's merely a chapter in your lifelong journey of health and well-being. The urban environment, with its challenges and charms, is a constant companion in this journey. Embrace its pace, learn from its lessons, and carve out your unique path in the maze of metropolitan life.

In essence, maintaining long-term weight in a bustling urban setting is a dance – a dance where you lead, guided by knowledge, powered by determination, and inspired by the success you've achieved. And as with any dance, there will be missteps and stumbles, but it's the grace with which you continue that defines your journey. The city's rhythm is your music, and with every conscious choice, you choreograph a healthier, happier tomorrow.

Final reflections and motivation for the future

In the heart of a metropolitan city, with its dizzying skyscrapers and a cacophony of life's melodies, our journey began. As we navigate this labyrinth, there's one undeniable truth that rises above the clamor of city life: Change, though daunting, is the lifeblood of progress. And as our journey nears its close, we stand at the precipice, not of an end, but of endless beginnings.

Reflection is more than a backward glance; it's the compass guiding our next steps. As you've journeyed through this program, each choice, be it the vibrant salads over fast food, or the evening walks over sedentary nights, has been a brick in the fortress of your well-being. Your choices, both the triumphant and the challenging, have narrated a story – your story. Own it, learn from it, and let it be the beacon for others setting forth on similar paths.

While it's essential to acknowledge the past and aspire for the future, there's unmatched power in the present. The 'now' is where actions transpire, decisions are made, and lives are transformed. In the metropolis, where tomorrow is often a race, harness the beauty of today. Each day is an opportunity, a blank canvas waiting to be painted with the hues of health, well-being, and self-love.

The rapidity of urban life can be overwhelming. And in this velocity, setbacks are inevitable. But each stumble is an invitation to rise stronger. In the shadows of these towering skyscrapers, resilience is your true north. It's not about how many times you falter but the spirit with which you rebound. Embrace setbacks not as failures but as stepping stones to a stronger, wiser, more determined you.

In our quest for the perfect weight, the ideal shape, or the dream fitness level, it's easy to lose sight of the journey. The path, with its peaks and troughs, with its lessons and discoveries, is as invaluable as the goal. The essence lies not in the weight you've lost but in the life you've gained. Celebrate the journey, for it has shaped you, molded you, and brought you to this transformative juncture.

Your story, set against the vibrant backdrop of the metropolis, is one of inspiration. But what lies ahead? A horizon teeming with possibilities. A future where each day is a chance to redefine limits, to push boundaries, and to carve newer paths in the sands of health and wellness. As you stand poised to embrace this future, let motivation be your constant companion.

While this guide has predominantly focused on physical health, let's not forget the symbiotic relationship between the mind, body, and soul. They are interconnected strands in the tapestry of our existence. In the days ahead, nourish them all. Meditate amidst the urban greenery, read, connect deeply with loved ones, and pursue passions that set your soul alight.

Your transformation, dear reader, is more than personal. It's a ripple in the vast urban ocean, inspiring countless others. As you step into the future, wear your journey as a badge of honor. Share your story, mentor someone new to this path, and become a beacon of change. In a city of millions, your narrative has the power to illuminate myriad lives.

As we conclude this chapter, let's raise a metaphorical toast. Here's to the tears and the laughter, to the sweat and the resolve, to the moments of doubt and the epochs of belief. Here's to you, the urban warrior, the beacon of change, the embodiment of resilience and determination.

The city, with its pulsating heart and relentless spirit, is a mirror of your journey. It evolves, it transforms, and it surges ahead, much like you. As the sun sets against the silhouette of the skyline, remember, every dusk is a promise of a new dawn.

With this, we don't say goodbye, but rather, until next time. Step forth into the world, with the wisdom of the past, the vigor of the present, and the promise of a luminous future. For in your journey, lies the heartbeat of a city, the melody of countless souls, and the symphony of life reborn.

Conclusion

As the final words of this chapter unfold, it's essential to remember that every conclusion is merely a new beginning in disguise. The cityscape, with its ever-changing skyline, serves as a testament to the power of transformation and the potential of what lies ahead. The journey you've embarked upon is mirrored in every sunrise that graces the city, reminding us that every day is a fresh start, teeming with potential.

The bustling streets of our urban backdrop have been witness to your evolution, reflecting both the struggles faced and milestones achieved. But, much like the city that never truly sleeps, your journey towards maintaining your ideal weight and holistic well-being is an ongoing saga. The tools and insights garnered from this guide are not just for today or tomorrow, but for a lifetime. They are to be revisited, adapted, and integrated into the ever-evolving tapestry of your life.

In this pulsating urban heart, you stand as a beacon of change, not just for yourself but for those around you. Your story, accentuated by each decision, every challenge overcome, and every goal achieved, serves as an inspiration for countless others navigating their paths. The symphony of the city, with its highs and lows, crescendos and silences, finds its echo in your journey, a testament to the indomitable spirit of human resilience and determination.

So, as we draw the curtains on this chapter, remember that the essence of your journey doesn't reside in its destination but in the myriad moments, lessons, and memories that have shaped it. Let the vibrant energy of the city fuel your aspirations, let its unwavering spirit bolster your resolve, and let its limitless horizons remind you of the infinite possibilities that await.

Step forth with confidence, armed with knowledge, fortified by experience, and illuminated by the radiant glow of your achievements. The city, with all its chaos and charm, is behind you, cheering you on, celebrating your successes, and eagerly awaiting the next chapter of your magnificent story.

Made in the USA
Las Vegas, NV
16 November 2024